TESTED

HOW TOP ACHIEVERS WITH
DIABETES HAVE SUCCEEDED AND
THE LESSONS YOU CAN USE
TO GET YOUR BEST RESULTS

Tim Hoy

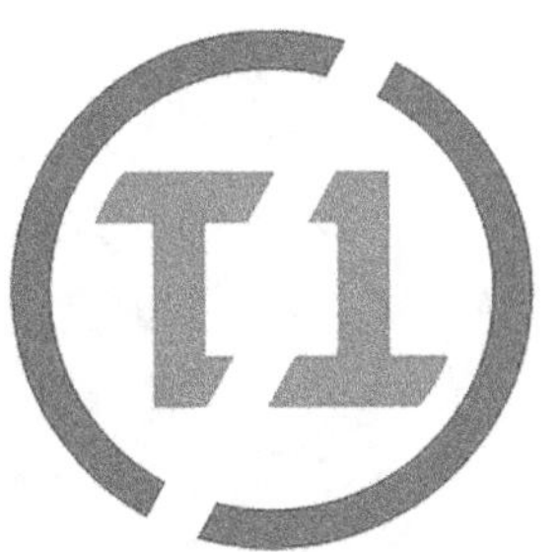

Table of Contents

INTRODUCTION

A master of anything has collected the most
mistakes of anyone.
—Anonymous

Have you or someone you love been diagnosed with Type 1 diabetes? If so, this diagnosis could be the most intense challenge you and your family will face. At first, you may feel overwhelmed, frustrated, scared, and alone.[1] But as time goes on, you will find that the lessons and skills you gain to manage diabetes successfully have many similarities to what it takes to be successful in general.

Type 1 diabetes challenges the strongest of individuals. Every one of the featured role models in this book overcame early feelings of overwhelm and frustration to reach their dreams, whether it be summiting Mount Everest, competing for gold at the Olympics, creating a business, hosting a radio show, or being a leader in the diabetes community. At times, they still face diabetes-specific challenges today.

If diabetes is not limiting you, then this book will add to your expertise and give you additional skills as you strive to life a full life. If you are struggling or are newly diagnosed, then this book will help you realize that everyone with Type 1 diabetes has faced a similar

---

[1] Of course, you are not alone. According to the BMJ (https://drc.bmj.com/content/4/1/e000161), Type 1 diabetics comprise five to 10 percent of the world's total diabetic population, meaning that worldwide, between 19.35 million and 38.7 million people are affected by the disease.

struggle. I provide some helpful ideas others have used to get them through the hard times, to succeed regardless of their diagnosis.

When I started writing this book five years ago, I envisioned profiling some remarkable people and sharing their stories to inspire those living with Type 1 diabetes. After writing and adapting the profiles, I realized it wasn't just the stories themselves that were interesting (as remarkable as each story is). Rather, it was how these high performers navigated both the challenge of what they were trying to achieve *and* the challenge of their diabetes.

As I dove deeper into each of their lives, I started to notice commonalities in their approaches and attitudes—the characteristics that led the people featured to become world leaders in their respective endeavors. These traits have been documented many times in books profiling successful individuals in the regular population, but never in those living with Type 1 diabetes.

The commonalities that allowed these individuals to overcome their challenges, move past their diagnosis, and fulfill a greater purpose resonated with me, so I set about reworking the entire book. I wanted to pass along the lessons that allowed them to achieve their dreams and aspirations while also managing Type 1 diabetes. I have collated their words (lightly edited for clarity) and expounded upon them with real-world examples to illustrate how Type 1 diabetes need not stop anyone from achieving anything. Whether you have diabetes or not, I hope that by examining and applying these core principles, you too will be able to achieve your dreams and aspirations.

Unlike other books that touch on Type 1 diabetes, this one has next to no focus on how to manage the disease or control blood sugar. (If you are new to Type 1 diabetes, the Appendix lists answers to some common questions. It is not, however, an in-depth discussion on how to get good control.)

The focus of this book, instead, is on high-level achievement, the specific tools others have used to become successful, and how you can use the same techniques to reach your goals while living with Type 1 diabetes. The success stories are about the journey to the top more so than the destination, so you can easily apply the ideas to your own life.

I hope that the practical, real-world tactics and techniques that these stars in their respective fields have used, combined with how they managed their diabetes in the process, will help reinvigorate your dreams. In these pages, I intend to arm you with everything you need to know to live a life you love.

The more I dissected the many challenges these leaders faced, the more I realized, surprisingly, that they didn't possess superhuman abilities. Their stories seemed to match other successful, inspirational people who did not have Type 1 diabetes. In other words, the difference between success and failure, or fulfillment and disappointment, was not the ability to produce insulin. Rather, it related to what these individuals decided to challenge themselves with.

Most importantly, these individuals seemed a lot like you and me. Before their successes, they simply had a dream or goal. They put a plan into place, took one action at a time, and didn't stop until they reached their goal. The superhuman factor appeared only after the skills were learned and the effort was put in. With some focused effort and application of the skills featured in this book, you too can achieve whatever greatness looks like to you.

Whether you realize it or not, you have access to the same skills as the people featured in this book—and you may already be using many of them. Some of your skills would be referred to as *conscious competence.* whereby you are aware of what actions are bringing you your result, and you can act that way whenever you deem it appropriate. Likewise, you have skills that you don't even recognize as being used, but they are helping you all the same. This *unconscious competence* refers to actions that are automatic, without you being aware that they are even part of your result. You're so good at something, you don't have to think about it, but of equal importance, you may not be able to leverage these skills on a whim in other areas of your life. Put another way, you know you are getting a great result, but how you are getting it is one of life's mysteries.

Chances are, however, especially if Type 1 diabetes is new for you and your family, you have also experienced levels of incompetence, where you know that you don't know how to do something, and you don't know where to begin. In other words, you have *unconscious incompetence.* We might say that you don't know what you don't know.

Part of the power of this book is to move you from unconscious incompetence to *conscious incompetence.* With conscious incompetence, you are aware of a skill or knowledge you are lacking, and you understand its relevance. At this stage, you know what you don't know—and what's most important, you can do something about it!

Being consciously incompetent makes you feel . . . incompetent! It can be overwhelming and demoralizing. The real power in these pages is, first, helping you to see that where you are struggling, you can improve, and second, inspiring you to make a commitment to do so. Others with Type 1 diabetes have walked through this process step by step, and you can too, no matter how long you have been living with the disease. The take home here is that the more you purposefully design the life of your dreams, the more competent you will feel, and the more you can go about achieving greatness. Diabetes just has to come along for the ride.

I hope you are still with me after that rather long psychological evaluation of the human mind. Even if that was a little esoteric, stay with me. By the end of the book, I promise it will be worth it. At this point, you might already have some cynicism in the form of "not another self-help book." I get it! But for the remaining pages, keep an open mind and try out some of the ideas shared.

No one knows your situation or the struggles you face, yet one thing is certain: the best place to look for ideas is from those who have gone before you. Of the people featured in this book, the age of diagnosis differed remarkably, from childhood to middle age. Some had family members with diabetes; others did not. Within this variety, I hope you find someone whose circumstance is like yours.

Break out of the handcuffs constraining many people in Internet chat rooms and Facebook discussions, and challenge any self-limiting beliefs you may have. Recognize the little voice in your head (yes, we all have one), acknowledge it for its "helpful" observations on why you can't do the things you've always dreamed of doing, and thank it profusely for sharing its opinion. It is time now to challenge your paradigms and move forward to the next stage in your life.

To be clear, this book does not provide a specific road map to success, happiness, and wealth. I do not pretend to have all the answers on how to live a happy life or master the diabetic challenge. That said, the tips in this book are easily applied in anyone's situation and are based on factual research. They have been given real-world bones through the profiles of the people I was lucky enough to interview.

Each time I listened to these interviews, I was inspired to rethink my paradigms about what was possible and refocus on my health. Having personally lived with Type 1 diabetes since 1976, I felt I had a grasp on how best to approach life. However, the stories of these amazing individuals reinvigorated my approach to my life and my disease, and I hope they do the same for you or someone close to you.

It's time to get to the real reason you are reading this book. What do you want to do? What are you telling yourself so that you don't have to start? Leave your cynicism at the door and try out the ideas in this book. My interviewees shared their stories to inform and inspire. The rest is up to you.

Now, make sure your hands are clean and your fingers are warm, as those featured in this book inspire you to test yourself. (Yes, the pun is intended!)

CHAPTER 1

MINDSET IS EVERYTHING

*It's not that I'm so smart. It's just that I stay with
problems longer.
—Albert Einstein*

When British Olympian Sir Steven Redgrave was at the start
line of the 2000 Summer Olympics' men's coxless four
rowing event, the goal was simple—win the gold medal.
This goal, however, held more significance for this crew than any
other team. If they could pull it off, Sir Steve would achieve a feat no
man in the history of the Olympics had ever before accomplished.

What feat was Sir Steve on the cusp of completing? By winning
Olympic gold, he would become the first Olympic rower to win five
consecutive Olympic gold medals. This accomplishment would be
even more remarkable in that the team would have dominated the
sport for 20 years on the world stage. As if this pressure were not
enough, Sir Steve had been diagnosed with diabetes just three years
previously. As he sat in his seat, mentally preparing for the race,
awaiting the starter's instructions, he knew that he and the team had
done all they could to make the gold a possibility.

As history now shows, Sir Steve and the British team rowed the
race of their lives, crossing the finish line at the Sydney 2000 Olympic

Games in first place, and cementing Sir Steve as one of rowing's all-time greats.

It could be argued that rowing had already helped to strengthen Sir Steve's resolve to take on new challenges. For those who are unfamiliar with the life of an Olympic rower, imagine months on end of getting up at 5:00 every morning to go rowing, combined with gym and ergometer workouts throughout the day, followed by much-needed sleep. The sport is enough to challenge the most motivated elite athletes in the early years of competing. The fact that Sir Steve had been putting himself to the test for over 20 years, and had been at the top time and again, shows the mental toughness he had developed before he was diagnosed with diabetes.

However, if we were to rewind three years prior to this history-making moment, then the true picture emerges of what Sir Steve overcame to win his fifth gold medal. British selection policy for the crew dictated that previous victories on rowing teams were not to determine current team selection. Individuals had to prove their worth in a variety of competitions, whereby those vying for selection were ranked against one another. For someone of Sir Steve's caliber, this process was second nature, and he was used to dominating.

But as selection trials began, Sir Steve was feeling at his lowest point. No matter how hard he pushed, he was just not making the cut. Naturally, this meant he tried even harder, putting his sudden thirst and tiredness to not being fit enough. Despite his resolve, his hard work was not generating results. Sir Steve was slower and more lethargic than he had ever been. Finally, he realized that something was wrong, and he went to visit his doctor. "When I got the diagnosis of diabetes," he says, "I thought my rowing career was over. I knew no one who was rowing at this level with diabetes. I figured, 'I will walk in there and hear the news, and that will be it.'"

When we look to our Olympic heroes, it is easy to think that they are simply superhuman, that few can come close to their achievements. What this story illustrates is that even the strongest of us, and the most capable, can be momentarily brought to a standstill with the same doubts and vulnerabilities as any other person. The difference between success and failure is what they do next: how the setback affects their mindset, and who they surround themselves with to support their goals.

As Sir Steve recalls, "After being shown how to inject [by Ian Gallen, who became his endocrinologist], I thought, 'At some stage, he is going to tell me that I can't continue.' Instead he said, 'I see no reason why in three years' time you can't be competing at the Olympics in Sydney.' Because of his enthusiasm and confidence, I felt it was worth giving it a go. He did say it wasn't going to be easy, but his philosophy was, 'Why not?' My philosophy became, 'Diabetes has to live with me, not me with my diabetes.'"

How does an elite athlete competing at a level where the difference between first and last is fractions of a second (and is often attributed to 99 percent mental toughness and 1 percent physical ability) manage the doubt and challenge of being diagnosed with a disease that no gold medalist rower has ever battled before? In Sir Steve's case, he simply took on the challenge and used it as a tool to learn from.

In her book *Mindset: The New Psychology of Success*,[2] Stanford University psychologist Carol Dweck sums up the difference between the two approaches humans generally adopt when presented with a choice or a challenge such as Sir Steve's. Some, like the individuals profiled in this book, have a *growth mindset*. They see challenges as opportunities to learn, develop skills, make and recover from mistakes, and reap the ensuing rewards. They believe they can improve, and they use each mistake as a chance to grow and make themselves even better.

Dweck describes the second approach to life as a *fixed mindset*. People with this mindset try to avoid the lesson by avoiding the mistake. They believe their abilities are fixed, and thus they never truly grow or enjoy the inevitable changes that life throws at them (Type 1 diabetes or otherwise).

As you are reading this book, consider your experience as it relates to dealing with diabetes—or for that matter, any other challenge you may be facing. When you look at the challenge, are you approaching it with a fixed mindset? Or do you see it as a chance to learn and grow? Being forced into injecting insulin, counting carbs (or abiding by other dietary restrictions), visiting the doctor, and taking blood tests might be an opportunity to learn how food, exercise, and stress affect not only your control of your disease but also its impact

---

[2] Carol Dweck, *Mindset: The New Psychology of Success* (New York: Ballantine Books, 2008).

on your body. Being diagnosed with Type 1 diabetes is a stressful and overwhelming time, but it also provides an opportunity for being supported in leading a healthier life. I'm not saying that you should be thrilled about having to learn these skills, or that all of sudden diabetes is the best thing that ever happened to you, but reframing the challenges can benefit you and help you grow as a person.

Sébastien Sasseville, the first Canadian Type 1 diabetic to summit Mount Everest, epitomizes this positive growth mindset and the impact it can have on outcomes. To give some perspective on what it takes to climb the highest mountain in the world, at 29,029 feet (8,848 meters), the following statistics should give you an idea of the magnitude of his feat. The climb takes place over a two-month period and is often accompanied by poor sleep, dysentery, and sometimes altitude sickness—which can be fatal. Winds on the mountain can reach a staggering 200 miles per hour (over 320 kilometers per hour). Climbers risk avalanche, hypothermia, and a multitude of bottomless crevasses. Once climbers surpass 26,000 feet, they are in the "death zone," so called because the human body is incapable of acclimatizing to the lack of oxygen. Stay in this zone without any supplemental oxygen, and your body is guaranteed to die.

The climb to the top becomes a test of preparation, mental and physical endurance, and courage. As of 2018, over 290 climbers have died on Everest, and most of them were in peak physical fitness.[3] One of these climbers was New Zealander Rob Hall, whose fateful 1996 summit attempt was chronicled in Jon Krakauer's best-seller *Into Thin Air*.[4] Rob, a seasoned climber who summited Everest five times (more than any other non-Sherpa mountaineer) died on the mountain while leading a climbing party. Seven other climbers perished alongside him. Krakauer's account gives context to the insane nature of this climb, and in turn highlights Sébastien's achievement: when the additional challenge of Type 1 diabetes is factored in, the danger is heightened—along with his achievement.

This pervasive danger was something Sébastien experienced in his own near-death experience. "One day I was going up a vertical

---

[3] Wikipedia, s.v. "List of people who died climbing Mount Everest," last modified October 30, 2018, accessed November 2, 2018, https://en.wikipedia.org/wiki/List_of_people_who_died_climbing_Mount_Everest.

[4] Jon Krakauer, *Into Thin Air* (New York: Random House, 1997).

ladder," he recounts, "and I went up 50 to 75 feet. There were three ladders tied together. I was going up next to one of the guides, and we heard a huge crack in the ice structure. We stopped and waited to see if the whole glacier was about to move. [Then] we just moved at lightning speed and got out of there as fast as possible. To this day, it was the closest I have come to facing my own mortality. It is something that I will always remember."

Sébastien's desire to climb the mountain stemmed from a trip to Nepal in 2001. After hearing the mountain calling him, he visited base camp. Despite having no prior climbing experience, he knew he had to try to climb it. He began to strategize on how to make this yearning happen. Life, however, seemed to have other plans for him. On returning to Canada, he was informed that he had developed Type 1 diabetes.

Instead of relating to this news as a dream-ending diagnosis, Sébastien was determined to continue his quest. Not born into a climbing family, or having years of hiking and climbing experience, Sébastien had to have the drive to do whatever it took to make his dream come true. Not only did he have to learn about climbing, he had to adjust his approach to accommodate his new condition. "I had to learn mountain climbing from scratch," he explains. "When I got back from that original trip, that was when I started preparing. I asked, 'What are the things I need to do to be able to climb Everest?' After being diagnosed with Type 1 diabetes, I found the first few months were difficult. You put everything aside, both your short- and long-term goals. You have to learn to do everything again. Then very rapidly, I realized with all the new drugs and technologies, I could still travel, and my dream to climb Everest need not disappear."

When chasing our goals, we sometimes think that we must be born with the skills or have parents who created the opportunity and desire to achieve. Sébastien's successful climb to the top of Mount Everest and additional achievements prove this is not the case. As we will cover later in the book, Sébastien used many different skills to overcome his lack of experience and stand on the highest point on Earth. What is even more remarkable is that upon summiting Everest, Sébastien then used the skills he had learned to take on new challenges.

He next competed in one of the world's most intense running races, the Sahara Race, a segment of the 4 Deserts race series. This five-day ultramarathon set in the Sahara Desert involves running 156 miles (251 kilometers) through what is considered the world's hottest desert, where temperatures reach as high as 122 degrees Fahrenheit (50 degrees Celsius). Competitors suffer stomach issues that they need to overcome, along with physical and mental exhaustion as they run through hard and soft sand while carrying food, sleeping gear, and other supplies. Sébastien, of course, also had to carry his insulin and keep it protected from the searing desert heat. The 4 Deserts segments are such an extreme test of endurance and mental toughness that *TIME* magazine has named them one of the top 10 endurance competitions in the world.[5]

In the face of these risks and challenges, Sébastien's philosophy to finish the race was simple: "When I do something for the first time, I don't have a time in mind. I just want to have fun and learn."

This mentality is a great example of how adopting the right frame of mind can make all the difference in how we experience a challenge. Your goals might not involve snuggling up to scorpions or scaling the world's highest mountain, but choosing an approach that gives you the space to learn from trial and error increases your ability to grow from all the experiences you may be having, both good and bad.

If being willing to start from scratch and experiment to create greatness is something you aspire to, then there are perhaps no greater examples to follow than Kayla Brown and Meredith Miller. Kayla and Meredith are co-owners of the Type 1 Diabetes Memes online community,[6] which was created to allow followers to express the lighter side of living with Type 1 diabetes. The page inspires and creates a positive approach to the many challenges of managing the disease by encouraging the community to make memes out of common diabetic situations.

Kayla and Meredith's shared interest in a positive philosophy led to the creation of this online community, which ultimately

---

[5] *TIME,* "Top10 Endurance Competitions," http://content.time.com/time/specials/packages/completelist/0,29569,1869820,00.html.

[6] The Type 1 Diabetes Memes Online Community group can be found at www.facebook.com/type1diabetesmemes/. You can also connect via Instagram (@type1diabetesmemes) or Twitter (@t1diabetesmemes).

became a business. They have turned some of the funnier captions into T-shirts that are sold around the world.[7] In so doing, they have brought welcome comic relief to those with Type 1 diabetes.

Kayla and Meredith were both diagnosed with Type 1 diabetes at age 20. Like many newly diagnosed patients, they felt a combination of fear, anger, frustration, and sadness. These emotions are probably not too dissimilar to what we have all shared as we have dealt with testing, injections, and constant analysis. The ease of a life without this focus was taken from their grasp thanks to a dysfunctional pancreas.

To keep some normalcy in their lives, they turned to the outdoor adventure group Connected in Motion.[8] This group brings people with Type 1 diabetes together to experience the outdoors in an active way. The two bonded at one of Connected in Motion's outdoor events, and Kayla shared how she had started a Facebook group based around memes of Type 1 diabetes. Together they agreed to form a partnership, and their Facebook page, which began with just 129 followers, now has over 70,000.

In creating a light-hearted approach to diabetic challenges and trying to see the funnier side of the disease, Kayla and Meredith have been able to improve many Type 1 diabetics' potentially negative experiences into supportive, collaborative ones. By approaching the partnership with a willingness to experiment and learn as they went, the two have created a remarkably supportive community, and their own skill sets have grown with it. They have learned how to set up an online shop and create time to manage the page as it has grown.

If you think you don't have the time to go after your dreams, then Kayla and Meredith show that you likely need less time than you think. They grew their business while they were heavily involved in attending university and learning about their own individual diabetes management strategies.

If you don't think you have the skills, Kayla and Meredith show that lack of know-how need not stop you. Neither had experience in online sales or marketing, but they asked questions until they found the answers they needed.

---

[7] Check out the selection at https://shop.spreadshirt.com/type1diabetesmemes/.
[8] To learn more about Connected in Motion, visit http://www.connectedinmotion.ca/.

Where many people go wrong on the journey to success is thinking that they should know everything they need to know before embarking. These same people also incorrectly believe that to maintain a positive mindset, one must be happy and positive all the time. When they can't maintain this level of happiness, they mistakenly revert to unhelpful self-talk such as "My situation is different" or "I am naturally a pessimist."

Contrast this mindset with Kayla and Meredith's. Perspective is everything, and as Kayla points out, this need for a constant positive outlook is unrealistic. "There are days when I get miserable. They come and go. You just have to go day by day and not let the small challenges ruin your days."

To be clear, many of us who have gone through a Type 1 diabetes diagnosis have a period in which the news feels overwhelming and debilitating. The difference between one person's experience and another's will largely be determined by the perspective each person brings to the situation. Using Carol Dweck's philosophy of adopting a growth mindset, a diagnosis of diabetes can be seen as an opportunity to make yourself an expert on what your body is capable of and how best to get it to perform optimally. Alternatively, a fixed mindset could be an excuse not to follow your dreams, not to become what you wanted to be—or to accept a less-than-ideal HbA1c because of your circumstances. (If you don't know what the heck an HbA1c result is, see the appendix for details.)

An approach that can be helpful in gaining clarity on this concept is to remember your childhood. You need only look at a 14-month-old toddler learning to walk to realize that people learn by making mistakes—and embracing them is where the fun begins.

For those of you who can remember learning to ride a bike, it probably started out as a scary undertaking. You may have needed encouragement to become brave enough to try again and again until the skill was mastered. The exhilaration and pride that you felt on the other side of all the mistakes opened up a whole new world. Yes, you probably crashed, cried, and wanted to give up, but the potential freedom it offered, along with encouragement from the right people, allowed you to push through what at first seemed impossible.

This childhood mentality applied to adult life can take you to areas you never dreamed possible, but you must start by accepting that you need to make mistakes to allow learning to occur. Learning to live with Type 1 diabetes need not be any different than learning to walk or ride a bike. Mistakes will be made; great HbA1c results are difficult to attain, but that does not make you a failure.

You fail only when you give up and decide the disease is impossible to manage. Your body is always changing, so what works for one day, one month, or one year may not offer the same benefits down the track. The key is to continue to embrace mistakes as lessons. Mistakes are not an indication that your actions aren't worth the effort. With each lesson you get that much better, and before long, your lessons make you a master.

What also differentiates those who succeed from those who don't is their relationship to mistakes and failures. Successful individuals (diabetic or otherwise) see a bad outcome as feedback that they may require additional training or effort before their next attempt. This isn't to say that the struggle to continue is not hard. However, those who succeed embrace the struggle as part of life's never-ending learning process and continue to seek out these sorts of opportunities to keep getting better.

Chris Angell was already on the path to success well before his diagnosis of Type 1 diabetes at age 30. He had completed a philosophy degree and an MBA at INSEAD, had started a not-for-profit business focusing on art works in Africa, and was working as a project manager with an oligarch from Russia who was that country's biggest exporter of Vodka.

To say Chris didn't let fear stand in the way of his dreams is an understatement. But with his diagnosis of diabetes came the challenge of dealing with regular hypoglycemic events. Worse, he hated the taste of glucose tabs, and it was driving him crazy. "If I had to eat one more glucose tablet," he says, "I felt that my mouth was going to turn inside out and leave my body."

Instead of complaining and hoping someone else might solve the problem of poor-tasting tablets, Chris took action. He began to question why they tasted so bad. On closer inspection, he noticed the product ingredients included petroleum-based food dyes and artificial flavors.

As we will see, sometimes our biggest passions quickly become full-time undertakings. Realizing the shortcomings of these products,

Chris tinkered with making a better glucose tablet as a side project. At the same time, one venture Chris had been trying to create with his wife was an organic candy bar business, but it was not living up to expectations. Rather than concede defeat, he leveraged the lessons they had learned to solve both problems. He successfully created a better-tasting glucose tablet, targeted at correcting low glucose levels. The company Jungell and its signature product, GlucoLift,[9] were born.

Rather than being a victim of circumstance, Chris took a problem in his life and decided to solve it himself. Those who work on developing a positive mindset see opportunities in problems, not obstacles in the way of taking the next step. You too can develop this mindset over time by asking one question: "What is the opportunity in this situation?"

I am sure that many of you reading this book have gone through the burnout phase; it is not specific to diabetes but to life in general. It is common to feel burned out by a situation that demands a lot of you. To give an example relevant to Type 1 diabetes, I have seen many parents frustrated because their teens have given up and are no longer managing their disease the way they should. How can parents effect a change of mindset in those situations?

The trick is, first, to have a goal that gives you a reason to keep going. For Sébastien Sasseville, it was climbing Mount Everest. For Sir Steve Redgrave, it was rowing one last time as an Olympian. Kayla Brown and Meredith Miller just wanted to bring joy and laughter to an otherwise thankless disease. These aspirations gave them a reason to find a way to live with Type 1 diabetes, to care enough to make the effort. The question you need to ask yourself is, "What is my reason why?"

At some stage on your way to your goal, you will have a challenge to face. Everyone does. Focusing on the individual part or the next step, instead of the whole picture, can make the situation seem less overwhelming.

An unhelpful mindset can work against us. With the diagnosis of Type 1 diabetes, some emotional responses can unwittingly sabotage what we are trying to achieve—even in those who seem to have it all together. Adopt the right mindset, and anything is possible.

---

[9] or more on GlucoLift, visit http://www.glucolift.com/.

CHAPTER AT A GLANCE

- *How* you think really matters.
- Give yourself permission to accept mistakes and slip-ups as simply feedback on the journey to mastery.
- Approach Type 1 diabetes with a growth mindset, one that allows for learning, rather than using the diagnosis as a reason to give up. Mindset can be the difference between success and failure.

CHAPTER 2

FOLLOW YOUR DREAM

Every pro was once an amateur.
Every expert was once a beginner.
So dream big and start now.
—Author unknown

If you are a cynic like myself, the title of this chapter might make you want to stop reading—or at least give you the urge to sigh out loud. If life were as simple as following your dream, we would all be living on islands, sipping margaritas as the sun sets. Upon awakening, with the margarita vanishing from your dream state, you can be left wondering: "How do some people have it so easy, why on Earth did I have to be the one who has to deal with living with Type 1 diabetes to boot, and more importantly, whatever happened to that margarita?"

But what if the idea of forming a dream isn't the problem? What if, instead, the process and the steps you are taking are causing you to fall short of the island and the margarita? In this chapter, we are going to explore just how impactful the dream life or goal you set for yourself can be—the difference between consciously creating what you want or accidently stumbling from one life event to the next.

When I first interviewed Sébastien Sasseville, he had successfully summited Mount Everest and was about to race across the Sahara. He has since followed up these achievements by completing seven Ironman events (think 2.4-mile swim and 112-mile bike ride, followed by a marathon—a 26.2-mile run). As if those tests of endurance weren't enough, he then set about running across Canada to raise awareness of Type 1 diabetes. In 2014, he ran almost 4,500 miles (7,200 kilometers) from St. John's, Newfoundland, to Vancouver, British Columbia. That's the equivalent of running 170 marathons in nine months!

Having completed these amazing feats, Sébastien now is a full-time motivational speaker and published author.[10] To say he dreams big is an understatement.

To understand how Sébastien arrived at this amazing point in his life, we must first look at the journey he took. Although his feats seem almost superhuman, achieved by a man tougher and stronger than us mere mortals, this is not the case. No, this man is simply a Type 1 diabetic who refused to give up on any of his dreams and in the process created bigger and better ones.

Born and raised in the province of Quebec, Canada, Sébastien did not start living with Type 1 diabetes until he was 22. At that time, he was completing his degree at Laval University. In his words, Sébastien's life has been lived in two segments—pre-diabetes and post-diabetes. Before diabetes, he was like most college students, drinking at the pub and studying for exams. Having this routine upended by a diagnosis of Type 1 diabetes could have changed Sébastien's life for the worse. Some would argue that the adjustment of living with diabetes is harder when living without diabetes has been the norm. The established routines that had been creating success are suddenly upended, and the paradigm of what life is like is forever altered.

As mentioned in the last chapter, Sébastien's idea to summit Everest started in 2001, a year before his diagnosis. In what he described as a trip that called him to Asia, Sébastien was already following his heart. Upon viewing Mount Everest, he decided that

---

[10] Sébastien Sasseville, *One Step at a Time: A tale of purpose, resilience, and determination* (self-pub, Tellwell, 2018).

despite his limited mountaineering experience, he would attempt to climb it.

Fast forward one year. This same person, with dreams of summiting the world's tallest peak, faced a new challenge that may have put his aspirations aside. The diagnosis of Type 1 diabetes halted Sébastien's plans and left him at a crossroads.

At first, it was hard—like anything new. As Sébastien puts it, he realized that he could not learn all there was to know about good diabetes management in one month, and nor should he ever stop trying to learn. More importantly, he decided that having Type 1 diabetes should not limit him in anything he had originally set out to do. His dream was to climb Everest, and diabetes was now going to have to come along with him.

As we will see, simply deciding to chase your dreams is not enough. You are going to face many roadblocks along the way. Some of these roadblocks are going to be related to having Type 1 diabetes, and some are going to be part of chasing something bigger than yourself.

The real key to success, I think, boils down to three things. First, acknowledge the obstacles in front of you. Second, find a way to get around them; anticipate them before they occur. Third, enroll others to buy into your dream and support you on your path.

With respect to Sébastien's challenge, this third key meant convincing the team of climbers he would summit with that he was up for the challenge and that diabetes would not get in the way or put their lives at risk. Summiting Everest requires every team member to be strong—who you choose to climb with can be the difference between life and death. To get on a climbing team, Sébastien needed not only to put in months of hard climbing training back in his home country of Canada, but also to show his climbing partners that diabetes was not going to endanger them.

Sébastien recounts, "The first few years [of training], I didn't look for a team as I had so much to learn. Around 2006 I realized I had learned a bit, and now I needed to find guys to train with. I went to a school that specialized in this sort of thing. I told them about my goal and dream and asked how they could help me. They introduced me to other guys, and we started to train together."

As he tells his story, Sébastien raises an important point: "I have always been public about my condition as there is nothing to be ashamed of. You want people around you to know [you have Type 1 diabetes] from a safety standpoint but also from a trust standpoint. I didn't want to be a burden; it is up to the person with diabetes to earn that trust. You do that by managing your diabetes as best you can. It is up to you show what plan is in place, what backup plans you have should something go wrong. To do this, my teammates and I climbed numerous times in British Columbia and whenever something would go wrong, I would have sugar to treat a low, a backup pump, etc. They knew that they could rely on me."

All too often, as Type 1 diabetics, we feel ashamed of our condition. We hide it for fear of being judged or excluded. In so doing, we tamp down on our dreams and aspirations. The rub on this is simple: if you want to achieve big, then dream big. The best way to get a dream started is to tell others and engage them in what you are doing. Sébastien didn't hide his dreams or his disease. I encourage you to do the same.

So, how do you find something that is worth your time and energy? The answer, most likely, is right in front of you already, and is probably simpler than you think. One of the best-selling authors of all time is Jack Canfield. The Chicken Soup for the Soul series, which he coauthored, has over 500 million copies in print in more than 40 languages. Canfield says that if you need something and it isn't there, then you were probably meant to invent it or do it.

Examples of this mentality can be seen in some of the world's most recognized and well-used products. Amazon was started in a garage. Jeff Bezos, its founder, saw the potential for books to be sold online and convinced his mom and dad to lend him the money to create what is now one of the biggest online retailers. Elon Musk saw a gap in the market and a demand for cleaner cars—and Tesla was born. Apple was the brainchild of Steve Jobs and Steve Wozniak. They wanted to change the way people viewed and used computers.

What solutions to some of your problems do you wish were available? Whatever it is, Type 1 diabetes should not stop you from inventing it or going after it. Perhaps, like Chris Angell, diabetes will show you a gap that needs filling. To further illustrate this point, let's look at two great examples of people who have put this approach into action, Kerri Sparling and Phil Southerland.

Kerri Sparling, author of *Balancing Diabetes*[11] and the creator of the blog *Six Until Me*,[12] is recognized as one of the leading online Type 1 diabetes influencers. In her blog title, "me" refers to Type 1 diabetes: Kerri lived for six years until diabetes came along. As an adult, she realized she was missing the connection she had felt as a kid going to diabetic camps. "After the diabetes camps that I attended finished," she says, "I had long periods of no contact with people living with Type 1, and I missed that support network." Kerri's boyfriend suggested she start a blog as a way of connecting online to others with Type 1 diabetes.

When Kerri started blogging, "there were only two or three people sharing, so I knew that if I was looking out there for a connection, there had to be others like me out there searching for the same info." Her blog was one of the first diabetic blogs on the Internet and has become a major force in helping people with Type 1 diabetes cope with real-world situations.

This desire for connection has resulted in book deals, regular columns, and speaking engagements. Best of all, says Kerri, "It has been a really rewarding career. I feel that my life is better for it just from being in contact with all these people."

Likewise, Phil Southerland noticed a gap that personally needed filling. As a competitive cyclist with Type 1 diabetes, he never seemed to get the specific focus an athlete at his level needed to manage the disease while competing, so he started asking questions. Instead of hoping someone else would fix the problem, Phil systematically brought a professional diabetic cycling team to fruition. The result is Team Novo Nordisk.

For those unfamiliar with Team Novo Nordisk, its premise is to find the world's best cyclists living with Type 1 diabetes, give them the support they need to achieve their athletic goals, and in so doing inspire and empower others.[13] The ultimate goal is to have Team Novo Nordisk reach the pinnacle of cycling by competing in the world's toughest cycling race—the Tour de France. "We have a long

---

[11] Kerri Sparling, B*alancing Diabetes: Conversations About Finding Happiness and Living Well, Kindle ed.* (Ann Arbor, MI: Spry, 2014).

[12] Kerri's blog can be found at https://sixuntilme.com/wp/.

[13] For more information on Team Novo Nordisk, visit https://www.teamnovonordisk.com.

way to go," notes Phil. "The goal is to get on the tour. By putting an all–Type 1 diabetic team in the Tour de France and making sure there is sustainable access to medicine for every Type 1 diabetic in the world, we can create a vison for all Type 1 diabetics to get behind."

Dreams can be big, bold, and intimidating. You must remember, though, that if you don't achieve the dream you set out to obtain, what you achieve in the process still gives you more than you would have gotten had you not started—and may lead you down a path you hadn't anticipated. Until Team Novo Nordisk, Phil had nowhere to compete with the support and specialized knowledge required for an elite athlete managing Type 1 diabetes. By creating Team Type 1 in 2008 (which has since evolved into Team Novo Nordisk), he was able to compete at a high level. As I hope you will notice in the coming pages, Phil's current vision is simply an evolution of a series of dreams that led to bigger and better things.

When Phil was a child, this process of one idea leading to a bigger idea began to show through. His love of cycling started at a young age, and not because he instantly loved it: "I got into cycling as a six-year-old. I wanted to eat Snickers bars, and I didn't want to wait two hours for the insulin to kick in. I realized that if I rode my bike, I didn't need to wait. That was the beginning for me. I went to the local bike shop, and the staff became like brothers to me. I started spending a lot of my time there. They challenged me and got me to push my limits. The great thing about cycling is that if you keep trying, you will continually get better."

Throughout college, Phil continued his passion for his sport and found it added an extra incentive to keep good control of his diabetes: "I was a swimmer, [I played] baseball and soccer, and it was very apparent to me that if my sugar wasn't controlled, I didn't do well. I wanted to win in whatever I did. If having a high sugar reduced my performance by 50 percent, then I wanted to eliminate that possibility."

At this point in his life, the dream was simply to be the best at any sport he could play. As Phil dreamed bigger, he shared his aspirations with others, so they could help him. Each dream and resulting achievement led to his next dream, and as the years went by, Phil soon found his true life's purpose thanks to a college course that required him, for 25 percent of his mark, to write a business proposal. Phil decided to do it on an all-diabetes pro cycling team, and the team now known as Team Novo Nordisk was born.

As with any project of this magnitude, there is a long road to get it off the ground. Before he was able to attract major corporate sponsors, Phil needed somebody—anybody—to believe his idea was worthwhile. This early support came from his lecturer Holly Colts, who encouraged Phil throughout his university project, and an unlikely stranger in a local Starbucks. After listening to Phil's ambition to form a team of elite cyclists, this random person donated $400 to his cause. To this day, Phil has no idea who this person was. Phil simply told him his dream, and the guy gave him the money.

This crucial funding allowed Phil to buy T-shirts, which he sold so he could attend Juvenile Diabetes Research Foundation ride events. Building on this success, he wanted to participate in the Race Across America, an ultramarathon bike race approximately 3,000 miles (4,800 kilometers) across the United States. He needed to raise about $250,000 for his grand scheme. Most people he told basically laughed at him and said he wouldn't be able to do it. "They said, 'You are 23, and you look like you are 16. Good luck.'"

But, like anyone committed to the potential of what is possible, Phil refused to quit: "I tried to network to the top. I knew if we could do this race, it could start something that would last forever. I got sponsorships from the cycling world totaling $130,000 in cycles and wheels, nutrition, etc. I was fortunate to get a sponsor early, and to now have the support of Novo Nordisk, who have really made the dream possible. Ultimately, it was because of Holly Colts' belief and the push she gave with the small snowball that got it all rolling. It is now about globalization. I really feel like we have only just begun."

As I am sure many of you have heard, simply putting your dream into the universe is the first step to making it come true. Naturally, it is easy to be cynical about this first stage. But phrased another way, by thinking about and focusing on your dream, you start to be aware of all the opportunities around you that could make it happen.

The key to dreaming big is simply to start. Kayla Brown and Meredith Miller's original dream, to add a little laughter into the lives of people with Type 1 diabetes, evolved into something bigger. These entrepreneurial women turned Type 1 Diabetes Memes into a business. Meredith explains how their dream became bigger than they had even imagined: "We saw a gap in the market. There were not many Type 1 shirts, and we have had an amazing response [to ours]. We just kept seeing the gap and responding to it."

Kayla was surprised to see their handiwork while representing Canada as an International Diabetes Association young diabetes leader in Australia. "It was great to see," she says, "that lots of people were wearing the T-shirts that we had designed and sold."

You get what you focus on. When Kayla and Meredith didn't know how to proceed, something or someone always allowed them to move to the next step. The outcomes they were getting were simply proportional to the questions they kept asking of others. This is a key point to consider if you are doubting the dream or goal that you want to achieve. You are not born with all the knowledge you need to manage complex situations like controlling diabetes, competing at a high level in sport, finding your dream job, or starting a business. What you were given was the ability to ask if you didn't know something, then try the advice to see if it worked. Too often we stop asking for fear of looking stupid. As you read this, I want you to recommit to asking questions and taking action. You need questions to take the next step toward your dreams, be it diabetes or otherwise.

Likewise, for Chris Angell, whose GlucoLift idea has made consuming 15 grams of carbohydrate a more pleasant experience, seeing a gap and not falling victim to the absence of a solution has resulted in amazing, life-changing events. Rather than writing complaint letters or whining incessantly on message boards, his idea has resulted in a product being launched and a business being created. He now also combines the skills he has gained to market Tandem insulin pumps. I hope what you are realizing is that starting is the hardest part. Once you take action, opportunities begin to appear.

In all the above cases, no one was born into doing what they took on. They just started and kept asking questions until they got the answer to get to the next step.

Ask yourself: what are you avoiding because you are worried about failure? Don't let your mind tell you all the possible negative outcomes. No matter how far you get in achieving your dream, simply chasing it down will put you in a better place than if you never attempted it at all.

In our next chapter, we will address the crucial step that is the difference between dreams becoming a reality or remaining just that—dreams. Dreams are a starting point to put action into place. For a dream to manifest itself into reality, you must focus on the endpoint and then take the necessary steps to make it happen. As you will see, hard work and perseverance are at the forefront of this process.

CHAPTER AT A GLANCE

- All big achievements begin with a dream of what might be possible.
- If something isn't meeting your needs, you should consider inventing it.
- The dream is a starting point to leap from. Most dreams fail because they are not backed up by action (more on this in the next chapter).
- You don't need to know *how* to do it, just that you *want* to do it. The world has an uncanny knack of giving you what you focus on.
- Dreams give you the reason to keep going when things get tough.
- If you don't have the answer to keep going, try asking a different question.
- Nobody is born with all the answers. Use others to help you get to where you want to go.

CHAPTER 3

PRACTICE, HARD WORK, AND PERSEVERANCE PAY OFF

There will be obstacles. There will be doubters.
There will be mistakes. But with hard work,
there are no limits.
—Michael Phelps

Malcolm Gladwell famously pointed out in his book *Outliers: The Story of Success*[14] that behind every successful person was 10,000 hours of practice. From musicians like the Beatles (who honed their skills playing in German clubs), to craftspeople, to working professionals, to the world's best athletes, successful individuals have put time and effort into their chosen passion. Sure, some were gifted early, whereas others developed their talent later.

---

[14] Malcolm Gladwell, *Outliers: The Story of Success* (New York: Little, Brown, and Co., 2008).

However, they all had the same things in common: practice, hard work, and perseverance!

Now, not everyone becomes the best of the best simply by practicing for 10,000 hours. However, anyone who does will be able to beat most of the world's population, who haven't put in this amount of work.

Why, then, when we are taking on a new challenge, do we expect to be brilliant at it the first time we try? Anyone who has spent time with a seven- or eight-year-old child can see this phenomenon when any new skill is being tried. The annoyance and frustration of not being the best is there for all to see, especially when the child is surrounded by those who have already gained the skill.

The question is, do you want to have the same reaction as an eight-year-old when you first start out? Or do you want to take a different approach? Realizing that a new skill takes time to develop gives you the space not to be so hard on yourself, to accept the inevitable mistakes, and to keep practicing despite the challenges.

This approach includes learning how to manage Type 1 diabetes. As a diabetic, from day one, you are now trying to learn a skill—a skill that used to be done automatically through your body's own pancreas. Scientists are still trying to understand this complex organ. The lack of a vaccine against Type 1 diabetes (or Type 2 for that matter) suggests that blood sugar regulation is one complicated system that has stumped the best brains for centuries (and despite online conspiracy theories, they have been looking hard!).

As soon as the diagnosis occurs, most people are overwhelmed—and rightfully so. Once the initial shock wears off, those who begin working hard on the new challenge begin to see the results (even if sometimes it feels like nothing is changing).

When Sir Steve Redgrave began to feel he was unable to produce the results needed to keep him on the British rowing team, he did not automatically know what was happening or how to fix it. He did, however, have a work ethic that made the path possible. He made it his job to ask questions about his performance and to learn about what he needed to do once the diagnosis of diabetes had been made. He surrounded himself with people who were willing to work as hard as he was to make it possible. As he recalls, "The diagnosis affected my consistency of performance. It took a while to get my levels right and to get my fitness to the right level. I also suffer from colitis, and it flared up again when I was diagnosed with diabetes. Every training session seemed to indicate I wasn't at the level I needed to be on the team. I prided myself on consistency, and I was no longer performing."

What I find most impressive about this statement is that Sir Steve did not look for excuses to give up. He was older than most rowers competing and could easily have attributed his lowered performance measures to age. He could have blamed his colitis or told himself he just didn't have it mentally anymore. Instead, he went looking for answers on how he could improve.

Shortly after his lackluster performances, Sir Steve was diagnosed with diabetes and placed on insulin.[15] He did not miraculously feel as well as he had before the diagnosis. Just like you and me, Sir Steve had a long road of learning still ahead of him: "I felt dreadful. I was put back on the medication for colitis and started to feel more human but thought I wasn't going to come back. However, as I came back feeling a bit better, I thought I should continue. After doing the trials in the single sculls, to determine who were the strongest contenders for the four spots, I managed to finish fourth. I proved to myself that even though I wasn't at my best, I was still better than the others. That was definitely a turning point."

Sir Steve and his trainers began to study this new disease—and they quickly realized there was a lot to learn. "Jürgen Gröbler, my coach at the time, researched all he could on the topic, buying books and checking out as many as he could from the library. This culminated in all the experts in all the fields sitting around the table at my house. Jürgen's first question was, 'Is Steve going to do any long-term damage by doing this?' We then looked at the possibility of going forward through that."

Chris Angell's approach is another great example of perseverance and hard work. Anyone familiar with entrepreneurs knows that four hours of sleep is common, as the rest of one's time is focused on growing the business. Chris typically begins his work day at 6:30 and fills it with procuring the materials for his glucose tabs, filling

---

[15] At first the doctors thought it might be the early stages of Type 1 diabetes, but now Steve is thought to have Type 2. His story has relevance to all of us living with Type 1 diabetes, however, as he needed to take insulin right away, and he faced the same struggles that go along with it.

orders, replying to social media, managing the facilities, spending some time for exercise (often surfing), and putting labels on bottles, all while managing his diabetes. I was exhausted just typing what he does in a day—I can only imagine what it is like to live it!

Through this hard work, Chris has secured many customers. Each customer is a result of his extensive travel around the U.S., visiting trade shows, flying on airplanes, staying at cheap hotels, and driving from city to city so that diabetics have a chance to try his product and in turn become believers. Many times, I am sure, it has all felt too hard, but Chris does it anyway.

I am not suggesting that to be successful at managing Type 1 diabetes, or your life, you need to emulate Chris's desire for success. You should realize, however, that at the start, you will have required reading, and challenges and mistakes will occur. That's why having a dream and the desire to make it happen are so important. When the process is hard, and you feel like giving up, the vision (which we will create in a later chapter) helps you to push through. As Chris comments, "I believe in the products completely. I get a lot of positive reinforcement from the community. I hear the difference they have made to people being willing to carry them around when previously they carried nothing. Hypoglycemia causes the biggest concern for diabetics, and what keeps me going is that I can make a small difference to this concern. The *community* also keeps me going. There is just this connection between diabetics. It is almost like you are meeting someone you went to preschool with. It is instant."

Hard work goes hand in hand with action. Failure to act is why some people have a book partially completed, sitting on their computer (could I possibly be talking to you?). Failure to act is why many dreams go unrealized. Once you realize that hard work and perseverance, not perfection, are the hallmarks of excellence, you can move towards excellence.

The reason why perfection is not a desirable trait is that no matter how well one does, there is always a way to make it better. An individual who seeks perfection will be left never feeling satisfied. Excellence, on the other hand, comes from persevering the best you can through the process, rather than focusing on the outcome. Inevitably, what you get is a great result, whatever that looks like. Embracing action and hard work over perfection allows you to welcome what is happening in any given moment, knowing that you are doing your best. Ultimately, seeking excellence allows you to keep challenging yourself and keep enjoying the process.

Take for example Jeff Collins. During his working years, Jeff hosted the breakfast show and later the flagship drivetime segment for the CBC, Canada's national broadcaster. While most of us lay asleep, this radio host resisted the urge to hit snooze as his alarm clock buzzed at 3:00 in the morning. He had to get to work so that others waking up could ease into their days with Jeff's voice keeping them company.

Naturally, hosting a radio show requires an amiable personality and an ability to connect with listeners, which, not surprisingly, Jeff has in spades. He attributes these characteristics to being part of a family of six brothers and sisters. Being the eldest of the Newfoundlander Collins' family, Jeff was no stranger to making conversation and handling opposing viewpoints.

Jeff's story resembles the stories of others who have gone on to live their dreams: he had a goal and simply took action. He didn't have a clue about how to get started, but he started all the same. On the advice of his mother, who believed that his teenage attraction to the stage would make for a great career in radio, he called the CBC's Newfoundland office as a high school student. He asked to speak to whomever was in charge of hiring and declared, "My name is Jeff Collins, and I would like to work for the CBC."

Jeff says, "I asked the hiring manager if I could come see about working for him. For some reason he agreed. We talked, and I asked questions on how to get in. He suggested I go to school and study broadcasting."

When Jeff inquired about enrolling in broadcasting school, he discovered he needed to complete grade 12 to be eligible. However, where he lived in Newfoundland, school finished at grade 11. "Rather than give up," he explains, "I went and did a first year of a degree at the local university and then applied to broadcasting school—and got in."

Jeff finished his degree and called the manager again: "I told him I had done everything he suggested. He then got me in at the ground floor as a radio technician. After three years, I ended up at CBC Toronto as a technician, but I knew it wasn't for me. I realized

I needed a portfolio. The news director asked me to put together a piece for a small radio station. I made mistakes, but after each one I learned something. That's how I developed my skills. I lost two auditions and got told I didn't have the CBC voice. I thought, 'I am going to have to wait till someone likes my sound and find ways to hone my craft so when the opportunity comes up, I will be ready.'"

Jeff worked hard at getting in the door, persisted throughout his career, and realized each step in the process of making his dream a reality. Despite not knowing anything about how to break into radio, Jeff simply took the necessary first step—he looked for advice from those who knew the process. He then took this advice and implemented it. When he ran into a roadblock, he stayed focused on his dream and found ways to fulfill it. At no time did he blame his circumstances, his education, or the people around him. He also didn't worry about whether he would fail or succeed. He simply started, and when the inevitable mistakes occurred, he used them to adjust and improve.

What makes his story remarkable is that he did not initially apply this take-charge attitude to his Type 1 diagnosis. Years after Jeff had made it into radio, and in his thirties, he began guzzling anything he could get his hands on, lasting for a stretch of two weeks. Having had a family member already diagnosed with Type 1 diabetes, Jeff realized that he was a likely candidate.

After tests confirmed the diagnosis, Jeff didn't have the storybook approach to managing his condition that you may have assumed given that he is featured in this book—which is one reason why I wanted to showcase his story. Our heroes have struggles just as we do. As you will see, his story should give hope to any of you struggling with Type 1 diabetes.

All too often, when we start out on the Type 1 diabetes journey, we are told that we need to get a low A1c, avoid hypoglycemia, and change our whole way of being. We can feel that perfection is never going to be obtained, which can lead to us feeling isolated and alone. If you have struggled or are struggling to accept your diagnosis, then Jeff's story illustrates that it is never too late to make a change. Let's dive a little deeper.

After his diagnosis of Type 1 diabetes, Jeff would rise out of bed to begin his long day and take just *one* injection of NPH insulin, which is a form of long-acting insulin designed to keep blood sugars stable when not eating. This would be his *only* injection of the day. For two years, Jeff took just one injection a day!

For those new to diabetes, NPH insulin is not designed to cover food eaten. Most people take a long-acting insulin (such as NPH) to control blood sugars when they are not eating. Once food is consumed, they will then take a shorter-acting insulin each time to cover the glucose. By Jeff's own admission, taking only one long-acting insulin shot a day was foolhardy. His A1c readings were well above 11, and basically, he was slowly destroying his body.

Things changed when he inquired about a study looking at retinopathy (eye damage common to Type 1 diabetics) and met Dr. Stuart Ross. Rather than lecture Jeff about the negative consequences of his approach, Dr. Ross thought about what might be most important to Jeff and his life. As Jeff describes, "He basically asked me how my sleep had been, which I informed him had not been great due to the many trips to the bathroom I made throughout the night. He then suggested that if I give myself another injection at night, just once to humor him, he promised me an uninterrupted sleep. Naturally, this sounded great, but it wasn't until three days later that I decided to give it a try. That was all it took. I was convinced, and I asked for additional injections to see if they would make a difference."

Jeff's stubborn resistance to his Type 1 diabetes was an attempt to live as close to normal as possible. Ironically, the opposite was occurring. He was tired, irritable, and less than his former self. Once he realized that by increasing his injections (taking action) and accepting the disease on realistic terms, Jeff got back the very thing he had being trying to protect—his freedom.

What message should one take away from Jeff's story? It is pretty simple. Jeff went after his dream of being in radio. He was consciously incompetent (he knew that he didn't know how to be a radio personality), and he just took action. It didn't matter that he needed to work in small town radio, do technician jobs, and follow the opportunity. Jeff kept the goal in mind, took the courses required, and never gave up.

Likewise, when Jeff realized that he needed to change his approach to his disease, he did not let his past lack of action stop him from taking it now. Admitting his shortcomings, Jeff adopted an approach of excellence in the moment to get his health back and ultimately his quality of life.

No matter where you are in your journey, your past dictates your future only if you keep repeating it. Phrased another way, the actions you continue to take produce the results you are always getting. If you are not getting the results you want from life, as we will see in a future chapter, all that is needed is to take new actions.

Sébastien's attempt to summit Everest living with Type 1 is a great example of formulating a plan and constantly adjusting as each obstacle presents itself. Mountaineering isn't just a matter of strapping on some ice clamps and climbing. It takes years of practice—just like diabetes. "If you are a basketball player, you will shoot thousands of hoops, so it becomes automatic," notes Sébastien. "Diabetes is the same. You have to train it so that on race day, you can be at your best."

Training makes a challenging situation more manageable. Type 1 diabetes has many uncertainties and risks—not that you need to worry, but rather, you must understand the risks and strategize to deal with them. Bringing this concept back to Sébastien's attempt at summiting Everest, the final push is the most dangerous and life-threatening segment. A well-thought-out plan is crucial. In Sébastien's case, his team's plan included his diabetes management. Everyone knew that if the diabetes plan failed, the summit attempt would fail.

Sébastien recounts his experience: "On the night of the climb, I worried. You are under a lot of pressure. You go in with a plan, but you have to make changes to that plan. Once you start climbing, you take a step, you breathe five to 10 times, then you take another. You have to do constant self-checks. Is it a discomfort, or is it turning into something dangerous? Do I need to change the plan? All that questioning goes on in your mind. I did my homework. I took years to get ready, but there was also luck and help from the universe."

Naturally, taking action is easier when there are few obstacles or little associated pain, but anything worth doing involves a certain amount of discomfort. So how does one overcome the desire to give up, persevere, and continually work hard when it all seems too much?

Perhaps Team Novo Nordisk's CEO, Phil, is a great person to ask. For those of you who have never cycled at a high level, picture your muscles screaming at you to quit, for hours on end, as your opponents try to destroy you. Elite athletes develop their own strategies for dealing with this pain. Phil says, "I just keep reminding myself that it's going to slow down soon. You learn to embrace the pain. Everyone out there is suffering. There is no easy way to ride a bike. I never wanted to lose; you just have to push."

Whatever your dream is, realize there are always going to be challenges and potential pain points. You will experience some failures and mistakes, but these are just part of the process as you get closer to your goals. By reframing the experience as a learning one, you will be among those at the top, who reached greatness one step at a time.

Perhaps the best example of hard work and perseverance being so important is raising a child. Parents often claim their children as their greatest achievements. Kerri Sparling is one such parent. Kerri, who was diagnosed with Type 1 diabetes at a young age, was left with the impression that being a diabetic meant her chances of successfully having a healthy child were low.

Of course, a lot more is known now about pregnancy and Type 1 diabetes. With careful management, there is no reason why anyone living with Type 1 shouldn't be able to have a healthy child. Managing the disease through two pregnancies has left Kerri with a major sense of accomplishment, in part due to the many challenges she has faced and overcome.

"Hands down," she says, "my biggest achievements were having my daughter and my son. I am humbled and inspired by them on a daily basis. They are far and away the best things that have ever happened to me. Pregnancy and diabetes don't always go as planned, but it doesn't mean that you can't do it. So often throughout our disease we are told no: 'No, you can't make insulin.' 'No, you can't eat that.' 'No, you can't cure it.' It is important to know that *yes*, you can have happy and healthy children."

Like Sébastien with his climbing plan, Kerri used all the tools at her disposal to reduce the risks on her children's health as a result of her Type 1 diabetes during her pregnancies. "I learned the power of a glucose meter and a CGM [continuous glucose monitor]," she says.

"The CGM was the most powerful and impactful tool. It put my blood sugar numbers into context."

Kerri had to learn many new approaches in her pregnancies, but she embraced not knowing and took action to discover the answers she needed to be successful throughout her pregnancies. Her hard work and diligence resulted in a greater understanding of her disease and two successful pregnancies.

With many variables and actions you can take, determining a first step can be overwhelming. How do you narrow down what to do?

Best-selling author Jack Canfield has some advice. Having had no previous publications and trying to get his now-famous *Chicken Soup for the Soul* into the marketplace, Jack didn't know where to begin. His early efforts to secure a publisher garnered only rejection letters, but he persisted. Rather than being overwhelmed by the thousands of things he needed to do, he simplified the task of getting published into the Rule of Five: do five things every day that move you closer towards your goal. For him it was such things as sending five letters to potential publishers, calling five radio stations, or creating five new marketing ideas. *Chicken Soup for the Soul* became an international best seller and a multimillion-dollar franchise. Any time you can persistently approach a problem with action, progress will eventually be made.

This concept is perfect for learning how to manage Type 1 diabetes and succeed at your life's dream. There is so much information out there and lots to learn. It can seem overwhelming at times. Break the work down into smaller, more actionable activities. You might start by reading five chapters of a book on diabetes (this one counts for an easy win). You could focus on doing five blood tests or getting five hours of improved glucose levels in a day. The tasks don't have to be complex, as long as their completion is taking you towards the goal you want.

Our friend Sébastien's advice to a newly diagnosed diabetic is a good way to end this chapter. "Go one step at a time, but always look to be learning. That learning curve lasts for your entire life. Don't look at it as a sprint, but rather a new way of life. Just learn a little bit every day. In five years, you will end up being a pro."

CHAPTER AT A GLANCE

- Persistence is the biggest predictor of success.
- No one starts out being brilliant at anything, but given enough time and practice, anyone can become a master.
- Break down big problems into smaller problems that are easier to tackle.
- Five new actions taken each day will move you toward any goal over time.
- Everyone experiences discomfort when taking on a new challenge. The more you embrace the discomfort, the better you can handle the challenge in the future.

CHAPTER 4

IT TAKES A TEAM TO BUILD

A GREAT LIFE

If you want to go fast, go alone.
If you want to go far, go together.
—African proverb

In the last chapter we looked at tactics such as just getting started, taking one step at a time, and using the Rule of Five to lessen the urge to give up. In this chapter we are going to cover the importance of others. When faced with challenging circumstances, it is easy to feel there is no point in trying. A common reaction is to withdraw from those around us and try to handle everything on our own.

An alternative approach, one that shows strength, comes from asking for help. As you will see, the interviewees featured in this book have surrounded themselves with teams of equally great people. For some, those teams began to form in early childhood; for others, they were made later in life.

Depending upon when the diagnosis of diabetes is made, the way we relate to this new challenge in our lives can be highly influenced by those closest to us. Phil Southerland knows this fact only too well. Growing up in Tallahassee, Florida, Phil was diagnosed with Type 1 diabetes when he was just seven months old. At that time, access to experts in diabetes management was restricted.

Thankfully, Phil had support in all the right places. Everything about his philosophy, both to life and to diabetes, he attributes to his mother's attitude towards his care. "I was just like every other kid. The only difference was I had to check my blood and give myself injections. My mother never said that I could not do this or that. As a result, I never had any doubts about what I could do. Diabetes was never a limiting factor. If it was controlled, then everything was okay."

His mother was ahead of her time. She insisted that Phil test his blood 10 to 15 times per day. Her primary goal was to ensure that by taking good care of his condition, he could prevent a lifetime of suffering. Thanks to his mother's guidance, Phil came to believe that Type 1 diabetes was not a limitation. It was just another obstacle life had put in the way to see how much he wanted his goals. This guidance is a prime example of how surrounding yourself with the right group of people can make a huge difference to the outcomes you experience. Often this guidance comes in the form of feedback, and not all of it is positive.

Humans by nature want constant positive feedback. Type 1 diabetes can be trying because the feedback is often anything but positive. However, as we see in Phil's example, feedback that tells us we are not where we need to be is important, and it can give us our biggest gains. The trick, says Phil, is not to dwell on it: "Great champions have a short memory. They learn lessons, but as soon as failure happens, they learn from it and then move on."

Research has shown that this mindset of embracing feedback—good or bad—and viewing it as valuable is the difference between continual improvement and stagnation. Failure is not the world's way of saying, "Give up!" Rather, setbacks are a chance to learn lessons and improve. Whether your A1c results or your latest performance review are poor, as painful as the feedback can feel, what you do next determines your experience of life and, in turn, your chances of reaching your goals.

Many businesspeople and elite athletes use mastermind groups to get through tough challenges and keep them accountable to their declared goals and actions. Group members offer suggestions and advice to help one another achieve their dreams. These groups work best when they consist of individuals with different ideas and opinions, along with firm commitments to achieve success. This framework allows for individual weaknesses or blind spots to be bolstered by someone else. Diabetes management need not be any different. Find people who seem to have their finger on the pulse. Connect with groups whose members are going to hold you accountable to your dreams and ultimately bring out the best in you. Find a mentor; go to meetups about what you are interested in. Bottom line, ask for help!

Team Novo Nordisk has embraced the importance of this concept. These elite cyclists are competing in some of the world's toughest cycling races as individuals, but they also work as a team and use race tactics to beat cycling's best. They employ the best doctors, bike mechanics, team managers, physical therapists, and team psychologists, each specialized but interconnected to get the best outcome. Each person plays an integral role in the success of the team, even though it appears that the riders are doing it all by themselves. With several podiums in the 2018 season, this approach is starting to pay dividends, and the goal of reaching the Tour de France is closer than ever.

For context, to be invited to the Tour de France, racers must earn their place through qualifying events and podium finishes in other cycling events around the world. These events require logistical management and funds for hotels, transport, bikes and equipment, team cars, food, chefs, doctors, sponsors, and the hundreds of support staff. Without this support, there would be no team of Type 1 diabetic racers on any of the tours. The team's results to date reflect the sacrifices every member has made.

As the principal sponsor, Novo Nordisk, a leader in diabetes care, provides funds to this amazing group of athletes and assists in getting the message out to the world that diabetes is a disease that need not limit anyone. Novo Nordisk also organizes meet and greets for Type 1 diabetics at every stop on the tour.

Too often pharmaceutical companies are the misplaced focus of many people's frustration with the disease. While I agree that the cost of drugs has risen exponentially over the years, this issue is more complex than companies trying to make large profits. Governments and insurance companies are a large part of the reason why pharmaceutical companies must charge the prices they do. Without the industry's efforts, innovations that make the disease easier to manage and financial support for those who most need it would not exist. By bringing awareness to the disease on the world stage, Novo Nordisk in turn helps in changing government and insurance companies' approaches to how they fund diabetes management and helps the public understand the difference between Type 1 and Type 2 diabetes. Through efforts such as these, the pharmaceutical industry is an important part of anyone's team.

Just like Team Novo Nordisk, Sir Steve Redgrave's story also has a large team element to it. Although his record of achieving five gold medals at the Olympics was specific to him as an individual, it was also made possible by many others, including his endocrinologist, his coach, his men's coxless four teammates, and—most importantly—his wife, who was also the team's doctor. Surrounding yourself with the right team means surrounding yourself with people who see your potential when you don't. Their perspective can pick you up when you are feeling down and help you formulate a plan to ensure your success. As the ever-humble Sir Steve states, "My success in Sydney was entirely down to the people around me."

This team approach applies to any situation in life. There is a common saying that the sum of the whole is greater than the sum of its parts. In the above example, Sir Steve's team stood beside him and advocated for him when he needed it most. Their support resulted in him getting through his self-doubt and believing in himself. Managing his insulin requirements was a completely new experience, and Sir Steve would need to master it quickly if he were to make the rowing team. There were going to be mistakes, but by aligning himself with experts, he set himself up for success.

Sir Steve says, "An international rower consumes 6,000 to 7,000 calories a day [double the average of a normal person]. We had to find an insulin regime that would control my diabetes with that energy intake." Ian Gallen, his endocrinologist, knew that the pre-diabetes calorie approach had helped Sir Steve to be successful. "We then set about finding how to fit my diabetes around this energy intake rather than trying to change what in the past had worked."

As Ian Gallen later wrote in a medical publication, "Steven's three years of intense physical and metabolic preparation following the diagnosis of diabetes, culminating in the Gold Medal he won at the 2000 Olympics in Sydney, Australia, speak for almost superhuman personal commitment and courage. This was not only a triumph for Steven and the expert support team, but sets an example to anyone with diabetes or other chronic diseases. With an understanding of how the body works in health and under stress, every individual can look to the stars and aim for gold."[16]

The team members who are the closest to us have the most impact on our outcomes. If you are reading this and are a caregiver to a Type 1 diabetic, your approach to managing the disease will affect what that person will experience later in life. It was true for Phil Southerland, and it was true for Kerri Sparling, the Type 1 diabetes activist and blogger.

When Kerri was diagnosed at age seven, her mother's approach made all the difference. She instilled in Kerri the sense that life was just as it had been before. The only difference was that Kerri now carried test strips, syringes, and insulin. Because of this philosophy, Kerri never felt that diabetes was a disadvantage to her. "I credit my mom with making my childhood seem just like everybody else's. My life wasn't any different from anyone else's aside for a few syringes lying around the house."

Her mother's attitude, and being diagnosed at a young age, helped Kerri accept the disease as part of her life. "When I went through the teenage years, like any other girl, my parents worried about me talking to boys I shouldn't have been talking to, staying up late when I shouldn't, and doing all the things normal teens did. The difference was simply those experiences were bookended by my parents asking me to test before driving and being more responsible if I drank. I guess the difference was that I was lucky to be surrounded by supportive family and friends who never really made it into a big deal."

---

[16] Ian W. Gallen, Ann Redgrave, and Steven Redgrave, "Olympic diabetes," *Clinical Medicine* 3, no. 4, (July/August 2003): 336, http://www.clinmed.rcpjournal.org/content/3/4/333.long.

A lot of successful people have this last factor in common. By surrounding yourself with supportive friends and family, the odds of achieving success are improved significantly. In Kerri's case, a combination of friends and family allowed her to step out of the shadow of Type 1 diabetes and never look back. But there is more to a good team than immediate family and friends.

Kerri's support was strengthened by a wider circle around her parents in the form of her health care team. This group helped Kerri develop the approach she possesses to this day and helps instill in others. "I didn't just decide that diabetes wasn't going to stop me. It was rather my parents, and my doctors, who guided me and said, 'If you are going to go out and do these awesome different things, then just maintain this one thing first.'"

The need for a supportive team goes even wider for Kerri, and she is trying to bring this message to the greater community. "I would have given up long ago had it not been the peer-to-peer guidance that I have gotten from the community. Peer connections are so important. They help you realize you are not alone and can give you ideas on what is available that you might never have known."

Kerri's words center around managing diabetes, but the same philosophy is key to achieving anything great. It also confirms the importance of one's mindset in determining outcomes. When Jeff Collins lost out on two back-to-back radio hosting opportunities in Calgary, he didn't give up. He looked, instead, for advice from his support network to help strategize his next move. "I called a manager at CBC Toronto for advice. She told me, 'The right opening will come to you. If it isn't Calgary, then maybe Edmonton. You have built up in your head a great deal of expectations. Keep honing your craft. Don't rush it. If you build it, they will come.' Fast forward six months, I ended up with a full-time job instead of a contract job in Calgary."

From a diabetes perspective, Jeff enrolled his coworkers to help him manage his disease while he was working. This openness allowed the team to help him when, on one occasion, he became disoriented and unable to perform a scheduled interview. They secured some much-needed sugar, and the show continued.

This point about disclosing your Type 1 diabetes to those around you is key. A lot of us hide away our condition for fear of being discriminated against or out of embarrassment. However, all the individuals profiled in this book have surrounded themselves with people who knew what to do in case of an emergency and who supported them in their quest to achieve their goals. By bringing Type 1 diabetes into the open, you gain the support needed to surpass any obstacles, mitigate any associated stigma, and help change paradigms of what is possible when living with this disease. Taking it one step further, it is against the law to discriminate against people living with a medical condition. In any case, I wouldn't want to collaborate with anyone who held a negative view of me simply because I have Type 1 diabetes. Don't be ashamed of what makes you unique and interesting.

Of course, there are always going to be people who are unkind, who make you uncomfortable for testing in front of them, or who miss the mark with their support efforts (we have all heard, "Are you sure you should be eating that?"). It is important to remember that these are small moments in time. By educating the misinformed to understand our condition better, you are making a difference for you and many others living with the disease.

What if you don't know anyone who can support you in your quest? What if you feel those closest to you are not giving you what you need? Then the answer lies in finding and asking for support from those who have been there before. When Chris Angell set up GlucoLift, he had no idea how to make a better glucose tab. There was no instruction manual online, no list of vendors specializing in such a thing.

Not knowing where to begin, Chris started by asking those who had already succeeded in the food business. He attended trade shows, asking the exhibitors questions on how best to achieve his goal of making the best glucose tab for treating hypoglycemia. If he couldn't afford the trade fair fees, he would look online at the list of exhibitors and contact them by phone. This is how he built his business from the ground up.

A common mistake you might make when starting to pursue your goals is to think that you must know everything there is to know. What successful people do instead is find others who are experts in their field to do it for them. In Chris's case, everything from packaging, storage, and order fulfillment is outsourced to those better equipped to deliver a quality service.

The idea of asking those who have the experience you lack is just as applicable to Type 1 diabetes. Chris has done a lot of work with the organization Children with Diabetes.[17] He was quick to mention that if you are new to the disease, the first thing you should do is reach out to those who are living the situation day to day.

"If I were a parent," he advises, "then I would for sure get connected with Children with Diabetes. The support that they provide in answering questions and connecting is amazing. One time a parent mentioned that they were going to go to Disneyland in Orlando and wondered if anyone else would like to come. Next thing, 200 families showed up. It is now a yearly occurrence. It could be also connecting with mothers on Facebook who have children with diabetes. Find the real people who deal with this to talk to."

For some, dealing with Type 1 diabetes can be akin to trying to climb Everest. Perhaps, then, the final word on the importance of a team should go to Sébastien, who faced the significant risk of dying when he finally summited Everest: "The support of loved ones and family is critical. Whether they like it or not, they become part of it. The medical team is important. Find an endocrinologist that is supportive of your vision. I needed an endo that would find a way. It is okay to shop around till you find someone good. As you get better, the team gets bigger. Surrounding yourself with others who have gone before you allows you to learn from one another. We can exchange best practices."

Whenever you are unsure or feel you don't have the answers, there is always someone who has gone before you who may be able to help. Go looking for that person—and more importantly, ask for help!

---

[17] For more information on Children with Diabetes, visit http://www.childrenwithdiabetes.com.

CHAPTER AT A GLANCE

- It takes teamwork to make the dream work. Every successful person has a team behind the scenes providing support.
- Managing Type 1 diabetes is made easier with a team. Having a support network to turn to when times get tough can get you through those tough times.
- Don't be afraid to try different team members until you find the best fit for your situation.
- Tell people that you have Type 1 diabetes. Yes, there will be some interesting comments, but at least people will get a chance to understand a key part of you and support you.
- You are a reflection of the people you surround yourself with. If you are not getting the support you need, it is up to you to find it elsewhere.

CHAPTER 5

OLD HABITS DIE HARD

We are what we repeatedly do.
—Aristotle

Ask anyone who is finding it hard to change a behavior, and that person will more than likely refer at some point to the behavior being a habit that is hard to break. Warren Buffet once said, "Chains of habit are too light to be noticed until they are too heavy to be broken." In this chapter we are going to dissect habits, tackling how to make good ones—and how to replace poor ones before they chain us to a life we never intended on living.

In a 2009 trial designed to assess how long it took to cement new habits, such that they were automatic, participants needed anywhere from 18 to 254 days.[18] The average number of days was 66. The take home? Habits take time. Different people need different amounts of time to make behaviors automatic.

---

[18] Phillipa Lally, Cornelia H. M. van Jaarsveld, Henry W. W. Potts, and Jane Wardle, "How habits are formed: Modelling habit formation in the real world," *European Journal of Social Psychology* 40, no. 6 (October 2010) 998–1009, https://doi.org/10.1002/ejsp.674.

Given these findings, it's no wonder so many of us struggle to incorporate a new set of habits when faced with a diagnosis of Type 1 diabetes. Don't give up too soon as the effort is worth it.

In the book *Stick with It,*[19] behavioral scientist and author Sean Young points out that so many of us start with good intentions only to give up later because we are conditioned to believe that habits are formed by an all-or-nothing process. If you were to change this paradigm/mindset and realize that change is incremental, that it is part of a two-steps-forward-one-step-back phenomenon, you could continue towards your goals without stopping at the first setback. With each misstep there is something to be learned, which can help make the next attempt easier.

Forming new habits as a necessity of a Type 1 diagnosis takes both time and consistency, with incremental changes and small improvements, gained from many missteps, which in turn lead to success over time. "So," I hear you ask, "what exactly does this look like?"

First, as discussed earlier, work out why this change of habit is important to you. Having a strong reason to do something (other than someone else told you) makes the effort that much easier. Those featured in this book all had reasons for better control, and their reasons varied.

For Sir Steve, it was increasing his performance, so he could win gold. Sébastien wanted to challenge himself by summiting Everest. Kerri wanted children and was motivated to share her struggles and connect with others. Jeff simply wanted a better night's sleep (hardly earth shattering, right?). Kayla and Meredith wanted to have a laugh about living with Type 1. As you can see, the reasons vary greatly. Your reason need not be world changing, but it does need to be relevant to you.

Next, proactively think about what might stop you from doing what you are trying to achieve and take steps to eliminate that risk. Remove tempting foods from your home. You won't need willpower to overcome the temptation, and you'll decrease the need to correct a high sugar. You might keep a couple of testers and strips at various locations, so you can test your blood easily as you move about your day. These are only a couple of ideas for illustrative purposes, but if

---

[19] Sean Young, *Stick with It: A Scientifically Proven Process for Changing Your Life—For Good* (New York: Harper Collins, 2017).

you really think about what new habit you need to create, a solution will present itself. You may have heard that powerful people have others choose their clothes each day and decide what they will eat, along with many other mundane choices. The likes of Steve Jobs and Barak Obama had limited wardrobes. Why? They weren't being divas: using self-control and making choices take energy, and energy is a limited resource. They saved their energy for the more important choices in their day. You should make it as easy as possible to succeed in your daily life by removing temptations and keeping things simple.

Finally (and most importantly), give yourself permission to make mistakes and then look at what led to them. If you slip up, don't give up because you "weren't strong enough." Instead, learn from the experience. By adopting this approach, the number of times you revert to your old ways decreases. The amount of time you apply the new behavior gradually increases. Before you know it, you will have achieved the goal you set out to do and can take on your next one.

Nobody appreciates the power of habit more than Jeff Collins. Getting up at 3:00 in the morning requires more than just an alarm clock. A habit must be formed to resist the temptation just to switch the clock off. But having been diagnosed in his late thirties, Jeff was having a hard time coming to terms with what was needed to successfully manage his condition. He didn't want to believe that much had changed.

It wasn't that the people around him were not supporting him. Many doctors' visits had focused on the importance of taking multiple injections. Jeff, however, just didn't think he needed them. For him, Type 1 diabetes was not as bad as everyone was making out.

I highlight this story because it shows that until you find the significance (or the reason) for making the effort, your commitment to do what needs to be done may wane. All you'll see is the hard work. Ironically, by trying to pretend that diabetes didn't affect his life, Jeff was allowing it to do just that. Once he found his reason to make the effort required, he took back control of his disease and improved the quality of his life as a result.

Incremental change is the key to moving towards a larger goal, be it Type 1 diabetes management or life improvement in general. In terms of his diabetes, Jeff didn't just wake up one day and change from one injection to five. Instead, he made the change incrementally.

Once he had tasted success with two injections, he decided to build on this improvement by adding another. Before he knew it, his sugars were under control, and he had moved from one injection a day to five. He didn't dwell on the terrible control he had in the beginning; he just focused on what was possible and moved toward it one step at a time.

Another way constructive habits help those on the path to success is they create discipline. The human mind is complex—just ask my wife! It gets fatigued by resisting temptation and making choices. When you set up your life to eliminate distractions that you must resist, you reduce your fatigue and increase your resilience.

Phil's philosophy brings this idea into sharp focus: "What it takes to be at the top? It takes a lot of work and sacrifice. When your friends are going out to party, you need to have the discipline to say no. That is where cycling and diabetes are similar. There is no one magic bullet that creates success; a lot of small things get you where you want to be. I have been far more successful in diabetes than I have in sport. The sport gave me the discipline; it enhanced my diabetes management. It would benefit anyone with diabetes to be more active."

According to a 2012 publication, people living without Type 1 diabetes had a mean lifespan of 77 (for males) and 81 (for females). By contrast, male and female Type 1 diabetics lived on average to be 66 and 68, respectively.[20] The good news, however, is that the medical profession has improved the care and understanding of this disease. As treatment improves, the gains people with Type 1 diabetes see in their life expectancy may be much larger than that of the general population.[21] A long life is certainly worth forming good habits for, especially when going after one's dreams.

Nothing covered in this chapter is particularly groundbreaking or revolutionary, but I hope it has made you take a step back and question what you might be able to eliminate or add as a habit to take you towards your goal.

---

[20] Dennis Thompson, "Type 1 Diabetes Linked to Lower Life Expectancy," *WebMD*, https://www.webmd.com/diabetes/news/20150106/type-1-diabetes-linked-to-lower-life-expectancy-in-study#2.

[21] Based on my Internet research, Bob Krause and Gladys Dull both lived to the ripe old age of 91. These two Type 1 diabetics would not have had the benefits of recent advances for most of their lives.

My advice is to choose just one thing you want to work on and make the change today, right now. What routines might make the difference for you? How can you tilt the system in your favor? Kayla's approach gives some insight into how simple it can be. She tells herself, "For 30 days, I am going to go after this project." Commit to your change for 30 days straight, no matter what. By the end of the 30 days, if you are now consistently doing that one thing, try adding a new one. By the end of the year, all things going to plan, you will have 12 new habits that are leading you to whatever it is you want.

The process may not be enjoyable at first, but with enough effort and commitment, great changes can occur. Most importantly, when (not if!) you fall back into some of your less constructive routines, give yourself a break and remember that setbacks are to be expected.

CHAPTER AT A GLANCE

- Habits take on average 66 days to become engrained. Stick with it!
- Incremental change increases the likelihood of success when trying to alter habits.
- Slipping up when forming new habits is common, but if you stick with the process, you can still have success.
- Habits lead to discipline. Discipline towards any goal leads to achievement.
- Increase your chance of success by removing temptations or obstacles that are stopping you from creating positive habits.

CHAPTER 6

MANAGING LIFE'S CHALLENGES

*You can't be brave if you've only had wonderful things
happen to you.
—Mary Tyler Moore*

I am sure that no matter where you are in the journey of life or Type 1 diabetes, reading this book may have elicited the following thoughts: "Great. These people have done amazing things and have overcome many barriers. But at the end of the day, they possess skills I just don't have and have the luck that doesn't seem to come my way. If they had my situation, I would like to see them deal with it."

You are right on one aspect only: your situation is yours and yours alone. No one is ever going to live your life. That is up to you. Trying to emulate what another person has taken on in life will never get you the results you are after. You need to find what *you* want to strive for.

Now, I am not one for patronizing those who were kind enough to buy this book and read it, but I have some thoughts based on the stories featured and my own experiences.

First, the diagnosis of Type 1 diabetes, the loss of a house, the death of a loved one, or a divorce all represent the loss of something familiar, a known way of being that was comfortable and consistent. It is human nature to mourn this loss. Elisabeth Kübler-Ross, in her book *On Death and Dying*,[22] suggested that people generally go through five stages when accepting such losses: denial, anger, bargaining, depression, and finally acceptance. The stages have no defined time limit, and the time in each stage is unique to each individual. When dealing with Type 1 diabetes, the trick is to keep moving from one stage to the next. To do this, you need to be conscious of where you are in the process and to acknowledge that it is okay to be there.

Second, as we learned in chapter 4, who you surround yourself with affects how you manage challenges and the resulting outcomes. People who have found success and are happy with their situation will be better positioned to advise you on what you could do to move forward. Don't seek advice from people who are at the same point on the acceptance line. Many in-person and online support networks are available. You must be careful, though, as there are also some negative places online regarding living with Type 1 diabetes, and spending time on these sites can prevent you from getting through the grief process.

In the famous Framingham heart study, which is the basis of the Framingham risk score (a medical analysis of someone's risk of dying from a heart attack), thousands of people have been studied over many years and analyses done on various aspects of their lives. After decades of research, the investigators have been able to show that if a friend of yours becomes obese, the chances you will become obese rise increase by 57 percent. (Among mutual friends, the effect is even more pronounced, with chances increasing a whopping 171 percent.)[23]

Based on these findings, I suggest that if you truly want to find happiness and come to terms with your diagnosis, you must

---

[22] Elisabeth Kübler-Ross, *On Death and Dying: What the Dying Have to Teach Doctors, Nurses, Clergy, and Their Own Families,* 40th anniversary ed. (Abingdon, England: Routledge, 2009).
[23] Inga Kiderra, "Obesity is 'socially contagious,' study finds," *UCSD News Center,* July 25, 2007, https://ucsdnews.ucsd.edu/archive/newsrel/soc/07-07ObesityIK-.asp.

surround yourself with those who are embracing life and seeing success. As the great Tony Robbins has espoused, "Success leaves clues." Best find those who are achieving great things if you want to find the clues for your own success. For every fan page on Facebook with people complaining about the hardships of this disease, many others are inspiring followers to greatness.

All too often, it easy to blame the disease, to let it rule one's life, instead of letting it be an accepted companion. What one person can manage may be debilitating to another, and much of this capacity has to do with the approach taken to facing challenges. Now I am not for a second suggesting that you are wrong for feeling overwhelmed (if that is how you are feeling right now). Nor am I suggesting that simply by saying a few positive affirmations, things will be all pleasant and nice. However, things can only improve once you accept what life has given you and you start experimenting with positive actions until you find something that works.

A prime example of the type of negative mindset that can derail your approach was illustrated on a Facebook post I saw. An individual stated that she had gone on a 10-mile hike. She had wisely packed her glucose gels, measured her blood sugar, and planned accordingly. After she had been hiking for a while, she began to feel worried; the time had gotten on, and she didn't know the track very well. She proceeded to vent on the page that Type 1 diabetes had robbed her of feeling safe while taking this hike.

Now granted, in this case, being concerned about the situation as it pertains to Type 1 diabetes is valid. The bigger question that comes to mind for me is, how sensible is it to walk alone in the woods on a 10-mile hike when you are not sure of the route and darkness is approaching? We can easily blame this disease for taking security and safety away from our lives, but sometimes this blame is just a fallback, hiding what is truly worrying us.

When life's challenges come your way, you can choose to blame Type 1 diabetes, or you can work out a way to solve them while living with the disease. Of course, that is easy for me to say. I am typing this book far away from your situation and place in life. However, your path begins with a choice and, as discussed, a mindset, not to let this disease get the better of you. Embrace the journey as you learn about what works for you and what doesn't. Type 1 diabetes will place many different obstacles in your path, and some might seem really unfair. The only thing you have control over is how you will react to the situation. In turn, your response to the event will determine your outcome.

This concept is eloquently summed up by Jack Canfield. In his book *The Success Principles*,[24] he presents a simple formula that I feel is the most important concept of his research:

The Event + Your Response = The Outcome

When an event happens, the only part of the equation you can impact is your response to it. In short, your response produces the outcome. If you are not liking the outcome, the only thing you can change is how you are responding to the event in question. If your A1c is not where you'd like it, what actions could you take to improve your numbers? If you are not fast enough or good enough to win races, what could you change about your approach to your training? Basically, the quality of your outcomes is determined by the quality of your questions about what actions you are taking to produce the result. Take ownership of your destiny. Accept that you will make mistakes but know that they will allow you to learn some valuable lessons.

Chris Angell's response to a challenging issue illustrates this concept in real-world terms. Many people had placed orders for his glucose tabs, but he realized he had a product shortfall and could not fulfill the requests. He was faced with a dilemma. He had many possible responses, and each would have produced a different outcome. What Chris decided to do was get ahead of the problem by reaching out to his customers publicly. He admitted to a process issue, which had created the shortfall. He offered to refund all orders that had been placed and informed everyone he would consider shutting the business down.

What happened next is a testament to the impact that surrounding yourself with supportive people and creating connections can have on an outcome. The majority of the Type 1 diabetes community rallied behind him and encouraged him to continue. As a result, his business survived a major setback and is stronger than before. By

---

[24] Jack Canfield and Janet Switzer, *The Success Principles: How to Get from Where You Are to Where You Want to Be* (London: Harper Collins, 2005).

managing his customers' expectations and being open and authentic, the outcome was better than he could have hoped for.

When Sébastien Sasseville decided to climb Mount Everest, before being diagnosed with Type 1 diabetes, he had no climbing experience to speak of. What he did have was a dream and the determination to make it happen. On being diagnosed with Type 1, instead of deciding that was it, thanks for the dream, time to move on, he took the challenge head on and decided to use his diagnosis to his advantage.

One of the many issues surrounding a summit attempt on Everest is the cost of assembling a team. The entrepreneurial Sébastien realized that many diabetic companies would love to leverage the challenge he was taking on. In the end, LifeScan (a manufacturer of diabetes monitoring equipment) supported the quest, and Sébastien became the first Canadian Type 1 diabetic to summit Mount Everest. He asked himself, "What is the opportunity in this situation?" and the answer funded his outcome.

Sébastien exemplifies the mentality of turning a negative into a positive, but he is by no means the only example. Importantly, as we just covered in the previous chapter, challenges need not be handled alone. Even the world's best suffer from self-doubt, but with the right support, anything is possible. Sir Steve was all but resigned to give up on his dream of winning a fifth gold medal. Needing to do well in the pairing he had with his longtime friend and rowing partner, Sir Matthew Pinsent, he started to think he was the weak link: "I felt I couldn't hold anyone back. There were three people who were world champions on my side of the boat for two places. I went to Jürgen, the coach, and told him I shouldn't be rowing with Matthew as I was holding him back."

The coach, however, saw the bigger picture. Surrounding yourself with the right team means surrounding yourself with people who see your potential when you don't. They can pick you up when you are feeling down. "Jürgen said, 'We need your strength. It may be your mental strength and the confidence you give the unit.'"

This belief gave Sir Steve the confidence he needed. Rather than focus on what he was unable to do at present, he focused on what was possible moving forward by breaking the challenge into smaller, more manageable goals (his response to the event). "Matthew said,

'We've got 10 days and we are 10 seconds behind the next crew. We need to find one second each day to catch up.' Every stroke we rowed in each session would make us that little bit better. It was more the mental approach than the actual possibility of hitting this goal that made the difference. We simply broke it down into manageable parts." Ultimately, by responding this way, Sir Steve Redgrave and Sir Matthew Pinsent made the Olympic team, and as they say, the rest is history.

Kerri Sparling gives those of us who are not chasing Olympic gold, or summiting a deadly mountain, the opportunity to believe that amazing things are possible if we take the time to follow our passion. We talked earlier about how she managed to have two children. However, in Kerri's case, this success only scratches the surface. In the online world, if visits are anything to go by, then Kerri should open her own country. Since November 2005, 2,909,117 people have viewed her site (at the time of print), a following that is larger than the population of a small country.

Rated as one of the Internet's Top 10 influencers[25] and as having one of the 10 best blogs about diabetes,[26] Kerri has won a legion of fans and is acknowledged as one of the first bloggers to talk about Type 1 diabetes. As one fan stated, "Kerri continues to be a wonderful advocate and spokesperson for people with type one diabetes."[27]

It should not come as any surprise, then, that when I asked contributors to online forums which famous Type 1 diabetics they would like to know more about, Kerri's name was mentioned time and again. How does a girl diagnosed at age seven end up being the unofficial voice of so many diabetics? Kerri attributes her popularity to her philosophy: *"If you are not pretending to be a know-it-all, then people can relate. To think that all you need is a glucose meter and some insulin, and this will lead to a perfect A1c, is ignoring the true nature of diabetes."*

---

[25] Riva Greenberg, "Top 10 Diabetes Online Influencers Named," *Huffington Post,* November 22, 2011, https://www.huffingtonpost.com/riva-greenberg/top-10-diabetes-online-in-_b_1096919.html.

[26] Hannah Nichols, "The 10 best diabetes blogs," *Medical News Today,* June 29, 2017, https://www.medicalnewstoday.com/articles/318189.php.

[27] Andrew Bell, reader review of *Balancing Diabetes,* by Kerri Sparling, posted March 21, 2014, https://balancingdiabetesbook.com/2014/03/reviews/. Bell has had Type 1 diabetes for over 20 years.

This philosophy allows Kerri to be both relatable and credible, which in turn are key traits of all those who experience success in life. Her online contributions are honest, without a filter, including such topics as pregnancy, dating, interactions with other Type 1 diabetics, and travel experiences. Through being vulnerable and sharing, she has developed great personal connections with many people.

When talking with Kerri, it struck me just how easy-going and approachable she was. When I mentioned the accolades she has received, she was quick to downplay them and point out she was just another diabetic trying to find her way in the world. This genuine modesty belies her strength. Kerri has not let diabetes define her, but in her words, it certainly explains her. Her response to feeling alone and craving connection has resulted in an outcome that is now her career.

"I was looking for a bunch of people who had diabetes," says Kerri. "I wanted to find people who knew what it was like to go on a first date and work out how to bring up the diabetes thing. I went looking for others, but there were not many voices to be found. I decided to see, if I put my story out there, whether I could find others in the same situation. What is astounding to me is that I now know more people who don't produce their own insulin than those that do."

Kerri was diagnosed with Type 1 diabetes at age seven. Like so many children diagnosed, the real impact fell on her mother. The regular ice cream sandwiches were a thing of the past, and a life of counting carbs was now the norm.

Naturally, Kerri has also had to deal with her fair share of challenges. Pursuing parenthood was perhaps her biggest one, as her journey included high-risk pregnancies, infertility, and miscarriage, and the ever-present diabetes. Even Kerri's health care professionals seemed to raise doubts about the wisdom of having a child while living with Type 1 diabetes, and the daily struggle struck her deeply: "The concept of *forever* really hit me. Diabetes is hard mentally. The reward for good behavior is another day of being able to try. It is easy to wonder why one should keep going. It isn't until you really get that by doing this day after day, it is rewarding you by avoiding the hypoglycemia and being tired from it."

What I love about this statement is that it shows how the challenge of this disease affects everyone. If you are reading this book and thinking that it sometimes all seems too much, Kerri's honesty shows that we all have these moments. Those who are succeeding in life keep going and keep trying.

Kerri's story also has relevance to this very important chapter. Part of taking ownership for your outcomes means you also need to take *100 percent* responsibility for the actions that are causing them. This type of accountability is infused into *Six Until Me*'s writing. Kerri is quick to point out that despite being an advocate for better diabetes outcomes, the voice she speaks with represents her own interests: "Anyone taking my word as medical advice really needs to see a doctor. Diabetes is so personal, and if you are not tending your own garden, then it will be sure to grow out of control. I haven't even worked it all out yet! I am just along for the ride, with everyone else."

To return to the original concept and apply it to Kerri's example, Kerri lives with Type 1 diabetes, and her response to it was to start writing about it (her actions). The result is a book and a blog that has attracted over 2 million visitors and has earned the respect of the online community (the outcome). What actions could *you* take to change the outcomes you do not like presently in your situation? Being accountable to outcomes is hard, but you are already ahead of the game if you are starting to look for ideas to change the experience of life you are having.

When reading these inspirational stories, it can seem that the people featured never had to struggle and that their sunny dispositions resulted in everything going their way. This couldn't be further from the truth. Each person in this book faced many obstacles and made lots of mistakes. Yes, they turned negatives into positives, but it was because they chose to do so. With practice, you too can make this a habit. Each time you hear that inner voice criticizing your efforts, try to turn the challenge into something that moves your life forward in some way.

Take Kayla and Meredith, for example. They believed the lack of humor and the negativity associated with Type 1 diabetes needed a different approach. Their response was to start a Facebook page dedicated to finding a lighter side to the condition. Like most of the people featured in this book, they haven't stopped at just one success.

Meredith keeps her outlook positive by surrounding herself with positive people. The death of her half-sister, who was diagnosed with Type 1 diabetes when she was young and who passed away when she was 10 years old, has had a strong impact on Meredith's approach to life. When Meredith was diagnosed 10 years later, she thought she ran the risk of following the same path. She used her fear as fuel to adopt good habits. Her half-sister really struggled with the disease, and Meredith wanted to make sure her life turned out differently. "Diabetes has such a negative air to it, and I decided it didn't have to be like that. That is why we started the page. Just because something bad happens doesn't mean you can't keep going. You can figure out ways to still achieve what you want. I never let it stop me."

Meredith has now completed a Master of Science in environmental science with a focus in entomology. She works full-time as a lab technician at the University of Guelph and is sequencing DNA for insect samples from around the world. Clearly, her being diagnosed with Type 1 diabetes at the beginning of her university career has not limited her focus or her achievement.

Likewise, Kayla, who was also diagnosed during her university studies, has completed a Bachelor of Arts, majoring in language and literature. She runs an Instagram account focused on finding Type 1 diabetic teen girls a safe place to communicate and share with one another, regularly blogs on her website, and is a patient advisor for the transition clinic at the London Health Sciences Centre in Canada.[28]

As they say, if you want something done, then ask a busy person. These two clearly show that with the right response to a challenge, you can find yourself achieving many great things.

We are not yet finished with the stories of these inspiring Type 1 diabetics, but to give insight into others who have lived with the disease and still achieved their dreams by being accountable to their outcomes, here is a short list of a few well-known stars. I would have loved to have interviewed them all. These and many other individuals are known more for their greatness in their chosen fields than for having done it while managing Type 1 diabetes, a fact that should resonate with all of us.

---

[28] Kayla's Instagram account is @t1empowerment. You can visit her website at www.kaylaslifenotes.com.

- Jay Cutler: American football quarterback who was diagnosed in 2008. Jay was 25 years old at the time and in the prime of his career He holds 14 Chicago Bears franchise records and made the 2008 Pro Bowl All-Star game.
- Victor Garber: Canadian actor who has starred on stage, in movies (*Titanic* being one of many), and on television. He was diagnosed at age 12.
- Gary Hall, Jr: American Olympic swimmer who won four gold medals before his diagnosis in 1999. He came back to win a further two gold medals at the 2000 Olympics. By the end of his career, Gary had won 10 Olympic medals.
- Nick Jonas: Diagnosed in 2005 at age 13, Nick was a member of the boy band The Jonas Brothers; he is currently a solo artist and songwriter. Nick contributes to many charities to bring awareness to Type 1 diabetes and is one of the founders of Beyond Type 1.[29]
- Charlie Kimball: Diagnosed at age 22, Charlie is a professional Indy car driver who, at the time of publication, has one win, six podiums, and 14 top five finishes in his seven years of competition.
- Bret Michaels: Diagnosed at age six, Bret was the lead singer of the 80's band Poison and is now a solo artist.
- Mary Tyler Moore: Actress who lived to age 80. Diagnosed during her hugely successful television show *The Mary Tyler Moore Show.*
- Anne Rice: Best-selling author of the Vampire Diaries book series. She was diagnosed in 1998.

---

[29] For more information on Beyond Type 1, visit www.beyondtype1.org/leadership.

- Justice Sonia Sotomayor: Sonia is the first Hispanic and Latina Supreme Court Associate Justice of the United States (diagnosed at age seven).
- The last person is YOU! I hope this book inspires you to do something amazing so that I can add your name to the list.

CHAPTER AT A GLANCE

- Make the equation Event + Response = Outcome your mantra. If things aren't going according to plan, simply change how you are responding to the situation.
- Our past mistakes need not dictate our future if we alter course and adapt our response.
- Life will always throw you challenges (that's how you know you are alive!). What you do with them will determine your result.
- Even when challenges present a potentially bad outcome, experimenting with different approaches will eventually lead to success.
- One bad day need not mean many more. Give yourself a break. We all have high sugars at some point, but we are not defined by one moment. We are instead made up of a collection of moments over time.

CHAPTER 7

ONE PERCENT CAN BE THE DIFFERENCE

*Success is the sum of small efforts, repeated day in
and day out.*
—Robert Collier

Forget large changes. It's often the little things that make the biggest difference.

With Type 1 diabetes, the amount of information you get initially can be overwhelming, and with the consequences seeming so large, you can be left feeling paralyzed. Any new activity, hobby (dare I compare Type 1 to something of joy?), or skill has many moving parts at first, but any good coach or instructor will break things down into smaller parts. Once each part is mastered, the coach combines them such that the skill is now learned. Before you know it, with enough practice, you have mastered what once seemed improbable.

Once you reach the top of your game, as any elite athlete or successful person will tell you, it isn't the 99 percent of your efforts that make the difference, but rather the one percent extra done consistently over time that your competitors simply don't do.

Chris Angell's work schedule is a prime example of this principle. While others lie in bed sleeping, Chris is already hard at work, planning his upcoming day and creating opportunities to promote his business. With only one other employee, a number of vendors to manage, and a limited marketing budget, it falls on Chris to make it work. Bedtimes usually occur anywhere from 11:00 at night to 1:00 in the morning, but when you are trying to make a difference and are passionate about what you do, these early sacrifices to generate momentum give entrepreneurs (irrespective of being diabetic) the advantage in a competitive marketplace.

When Chris elaborates on his work day, it becomes apparent to me that smaller actions done consistently are enabling him to challenge the bigger companies and ultimately bring his product to market. His days center around a combination of traveling to conferences to get the word out about his product, answering consumer emails, coordinating the vendors that help put the product together, and solving the inevitable problems that come up. He also allows for time to take care of his health by doing 20 minutes of exercise. No one effort has allowed him to get to this point, but rather a collection of small efforts applied consistently towards his goal. If that wasn't enough, Chris is also a marketer for the Tandem insulin pump company!

When people are first diagnosed, it is hard to think of where to even begin. Chris's one percent suggestion might provide some help: "I think you should start reading things right away. It doesn't matter what you read; it isn't about finding the answers, but rather what things you want to be concerned with. It should be a way of starting to formulate questions around the topics you are reading. Don't try to figure it all out and solve an unsolvable problem. Rather, find some questions that, if answered, will make the process that much easier."

One percent extra effort applied over a year adds up to a difference of 365 percent. The combination of doing one percent more and not giving up is the secret to achieving your goals in life. This same rule of thumb can be applied to learning a new skill. If every day you were to learn something new about Type 1 diabetes, before long, that one percent extra would make you a master. Likewise, if you want to start a business or take on a challenge you never thought possible, doing one percent extra every day will eventually lead you to your goal.

Sir Steve's early morning starts, followed by many hours in the gym, and his focus on learning how to make his body perform at its best while living with diabetes exemplify this concept. Sure, he had some natural talent, but so have many others who have competed at this level. The difference to his performance and understanding of his body was simply the extra one percent he put in every day. Not only did it put him on the Olympic team—ultimately it secured him his fifth consecutive gold medal at the 2000 Sydney Olympic Games.

When it comes to elite sports, Phil Southerland, cofounder and CEO of Team Novo Nordisk, can relate to Sir Steve's experience. Cycling hundreds of kilometers on the edge of exhaustion involves a large amount of training and commitment. One does not simply go for a ride around the neighborhood and then declare oneself ready to compete in the Race Across America, let alone manage the challenge of diabetes (no matter how many Snickers bars you want to eat). But Phil and his fellow Type 1 diabetic teammate Joe Eldridge decided this crazy event was something they needed to take on.

The Race Across America is one of the toughest ultra-endurance races in the world. Competitors start in California and finish on the east coast. This route makes the race longer than the Tour de France. As if that isn't enough, the race is on until teams cross the finish line. That rule means sleep is only an option, as is stopping for meal breaks. The race is definitely not your Sunday ride!

To compete to win with his team, Phil had to incrementally increase his endurance and his mental toughness. His approach led to Eldridge and him placing second in 2006 and going on to win the 2007 team event in an amazing time of 5 days, 16 hours, and 4 minutes. In the following years, with some additional Type 1 riders, they won the 2009 and 2010 team events. The journey each time took them over 3,000 miles and put the Type 1 diabetic team on the map as a real force in cycling.

In a lot of ways, Phil says, racing has similarities to managing Type 1 diabetes. "Diabetes and cycling are very similar. There is no one magic bullet that creates success. There are a lot of small things that you can do that can incrementally get you to where you want to be. Maybe it's checking your blood glucose more, maybe it is giving your insulin before meals instead of after meals, maybe it's eating a little better diet. It is a discipline. That discipline helped me in the sport I competed in, and likewise, the sport enhanced my diabetes management."

Ultimately, the commitment to these incremental gains leads to success, and the process continues to deliver for Phil. In 2018 he won the 60-mile Fools Gold Mountain Bike Race. As he notes, "The great thing about cycling is that as long as you keep trying, you will continually get better. So, I kept trying, and I kept getting better." Apply this thinking to your diabetes management, or the next goal you are trying to achieve, and no matter what, you will end up further ahead than before you started.

Let's bring this discussion back to you. For most of you reading this book, the information overload that occurs when learning about Type 1 diabetes is significant. Research indicates that the most information someone can successfully process and remember at one time is three to five pieces. Just try to remember the names of more than five people you meet for the first time at a party. This challenge of remembering new information—and a lot of it—makes learning about diabetes overwhelming.

So, what can you do to make it easier?

When learning any new skill, the best option is to break down the totality of the information into smaller chunks. As the famous saying goes, "Rome was not built in a day," and neither is the mastery of Type 1 diabetes. All the people featured in this book came to terms with the management of their disease state over a longer period of time and achieved their goals in life with a similar approach. It pays to remember that you are not born with the ability to "think like a pancreas." Diabetes management is a learned skill, like walking, talking, or riding a bike. Nor are you born with the ability to write a book, compete in a sport, create a business, or amass a following online. Once you accept that life is a process of continual learning, and that everyone starts from the same place, you are in a position to take the first step—starting.

Burnout often occurs in managing diabetes. Whether you are new to Type 1 diabetes or have had it a long time, the demands of the disease involve a lot of preparation and monitoring. From the moment you get up to the minute you go to bed, you must always be making corrections, testing, giving insulin, considering what food to eat, and timing your consumption of it. Of course, this lifestyle is not foreign to you, and you don't need me to belabor the point. What is interesting, though, is that this process can be physically and emotionally taxing and can become a major part of what you think about and act upon during your waking hours.

In *The Organized Mind*, Daniel J. Levitin[30] collates a number of practical tips related to neuroscience that might help make the necessities of this disease less tiresome. Levitin's first point is that multitasking is a fallacy. If you don't dump tasks related to diabetes onto a to-do list, the brain attempts to remember everything, taking over your thoughts of the day. As a result, you become exhausted as you also try to keep other important nondiabetic tasks in your working memory.

Not having critical bodily functions happen automatically can cause a lot of stress. This is one of the reasons many individuals newly diagnosed with any disease find it so overwhelming and frustrating. By making treatment a habit, the task does not consume so much brainpower, and disease management becomes easier. This process is akin to learning to drive a car. When you first hop in, everything seems foreign. There are so many buttons and procedures that need to be done in a certain order before you even put the car in gear. But in time, these steps become automatic (hopefully without dinging the car!). You eventually get to the point that you don't even have to think about them—unconscious competence. This should be where you are trying to get to with your Type 1 diabetes management and with any skill you are trying to develop. Expect it to start out hard but know it will get easier. Write the tasks down to minimize the energy required to remember them while you are learning to make them automatic.

Surprisingly (and I am sorry to break it to all you "expert" multitaskers out there), Levitin illustrates that working on multiple tasks at once yields worse results than if you separately give each task your full, undivided attention. This finding might explain why, as we get more experienced at giving insulin at mealtimes, while we're

---

[30] Daniel J. Levitin, *The Organized Mind: Thinking Straight in the Age of Information Overload* (Toronto: Penguin Canada, 2014).

doing other things, the recollection of whether we gave our insulin or tested our blood gets a little blurry (something I can attest to, as the most referenced menu item on my pump is the history option).

Looking for practical tips to help in this manner? To paraphrase the work of Levitin (and others), many one percent changes can simplify the process.

1. Write down a to-do list for the day. This list, for the record, should include all important tasks, not just those limited to Type 1 diabetes. If the doctor said, "For the next three weeks, I need you to be conducting an extra test after dinner," do not tax the brain with the task of remembering. Instead, write it down. This act frees up your mind for other important initiatives and gives your brain a chance to recuperate.

2. Have a place for everything. As we can all attest, looking for diabetic supplies and the car keys can really add to the extra time we waste on tasks. Once again, our neuroscientist friend has some suggestions. By consistently placing testers and insulin supplies in the same spot, you no longer have to focus on where they are. The same goes for car keys. By allocating a specific area to place them each time you enter the house, you reduce the chances of spending endless hours searching for where you put them.

Likewise, if you are going on a holiday, place the supplies you need in the same area of your bag and in the same area of your accommodation to reduce the likelihood of missing the opportunity to suntan because you cannot find your test strips (or for that matter your passport). With the extra time you save not looking for these items, you will no longer have the excuse that you do not have the time to pursue your aspirations. Time to get started!

3. Filing systems help. Another helpful tip that applies not to just Type 1 diabetes, but to anything related to life, is establishing a great filing system. While some of you might utilize my old technique of "F for Floor," having your documents easily accessible makes the time and stress of trying to find relevant information, and therefore your experience of living with Type 1 diabetes, a much more enjoyable experience. Now, admittedly, I need to redo my system soon, and when you first make the effort it is time consuming. But it will really make a difference to finding documents easily, when you need them, provided you put in the time upfront to create the system. Not to mention, your office will look a lot tidier—bonus!

On first being diagnosed, creating a Type 1 diabetes folder as a starting point would be a great idea. Then, as time goes on, take the extra step of making subfolders within the folder. If any of these subfolders has more than 50 pages, consider making an additional subfolder, lowering the page count to a more manageable number. You may have subfolder titles such as (but by no means limited to) "diabetes device instruction manuals," "medical insurance claims," "claimable tax items," "medical letters," and even "diabetes resources." If you were to apply this idea to the rest of your paperwork strewn throughout your house, you would be living in organized bliss. I know my wife certainly likes it when I take the time to do it (she also wishes I did it more)!

4. Use a planner and plan your time. Keeping on top of the many demands on your time can be a real chore. Your job, your studies, your children's needs (if you have them), and now the demands of appointments related to your Type 1 diabetes (or your significant other's appointments) can be a pain. However, if you were to apply some of the lessons learned by Fortune 500 executive assistants, you could make the brain drain related to organizing and remembering all of these important commitments a little less taxing.

First, if you do not own a planner, get one.

If you already own a planner, then make sure you are getting the most out of it. Writing down appointments is one thing; however, taking the extra step to remind yourself in the planner of what is required as preparation will be a huge asset. Examples of this one percent more include reminding yourself to get your HbA1c tested a week before visiting your endocrinologist or to get the printout of your glucose meter's results two weeks beforehand. This foresight will make it more likely you will turn up with something to talk about with your health care team, so they can really make a difference to your outcomes.

This same concept applied to your life will allow you to be more deliberate in your approach to achieving your goals. For example, prior to holidays, set a reminder two weeks before your departure date to arrange for extra supplies to be gathered from the pharmacy, leaving you enough time to see the doctor if for some reason there is a problem with your prescription.

If you want to get to the level of those who have achieved their dreams, allocate your time. Sir Steve would have a schedule leading up to the Olympics. He knew what he had to do at any given point of the day and allocated his time to that specific task. Chris Angell does not randomly run his business on the whim of the moment. He has a focus that starts with his planner, allocating his time depending on the needs he is trying to address.

Likewise, when Sébastien was attempting to summit Everest, he may not have had a paper planner in his tent, but he certainly had a plan as to when he had to be out of his tent and on the mountain. Each moment was meticulously planned to make the most of the weather conditions and the time needed to acclimatize at each level of the mountain. Failure to plan would have increased the chances of disaster exponentially.

Meredith and Kayla both allocate specific time to ensure that their Type 1 Diabetes Memes online community is updated, that orders for the T-shirts have gone out, and that they are replying to questions and queries. They plan around the many other demands on their time, which include running other individual websites, engaging in social activities, and working their full-time jobs.

5. Make the most of your technology—whatever it is. What has been the most fascinating aspect of interviewing these amazingly busy and successful individuals is that nobody approached their condition the same way. One would think that an Olympic athlete would have been all over new technology. Surprisingly, although Sir Steve now uses an insulin pump and a continuous glucose monitor to help control his diabetes, he was using older insulin and regular testing when he won his fifth Olympic gold medal at the 2000 Sydney Olympic Games. What made the difference for good control in his gold medal quest was not his technology, but rather the methodical approach he followed with what was available at the time.

Chris Angell's demanding entrepreneurial lifestyle was managed by multiple daily injections for the first few years. He incorporated an insulin pump well after he had been using a continuous glucose monitor to try to manage the ups and downs and related stressors. When food technology was not meeting his needs, he acted and created his own in the form of GlucoLift.

What about summiting Everest? Surely one must have the latest and greatest to have half a shot at success. The opposite turns out to be true. Given that no recent technology had been tested or used above a certain altitude, Sébastien was unable to test accurately. Even though he was on a pump, he had to supplement it with backup injections in order to summit. The point is that this challenge did not stop him. Instead, he did one percent more to overcome the challenge: "I climbed Everest with a pump. All the glucose monitors and pumps were approved to 10,000 feet [Everest is 29,029 feet]. I tested them above 10,000 feet in previous climbs. The glucose monitors above those levels become very inaccurate. We didn't know about the [accuracy of the] pump, so I carried insulin pens so even if it malfunctioned, I could still climb. In normal situations, good control is very important to me, but for these small moments in time, in order to stay safe, I am not looking for an A1c of 7. Likewise, I do not want to go into DKA [diabetic ketoacidosis]. It is simply, what puts me in the best position to achieve the goal of summiting Everest?"

If anything, the stories throughout this book prove that as much as technology can make Type 1 diabetes management a lot easier, not having access to the latest and greatest should not mean you cannot achieve your dreams. What you can control is getting to know your body with the technology at your disposal. This idea is just as relevant at sea level as it was at high altitude for Sébastien: "At very high altitudes, testing was next to impossible. You could test three times in a row and get a different result each time. What was important was getting to know my body so well that I was not as reliant on the results from the meter. It became all about safety."

Similarly, Phil Southerland did not ride with a pump or a continuous glucose monitor when he was competing. Instead, he learned to listen to what his body was telling him. Cyclists on road races push themselves to the limit of physical endurance over hundreds of miles. The exercise itself causes glucose to be absorbed quickly due to the large muscle groups involved, moving the glucose out of the bloodstream and into the cells that need it. Riders will often ride at just 10 percent of their normal basal rates and need to supplement this baseline by ingesting carbohydrates throughout the race. Phil didn't just ride by the seat of his pants (pun intended); he took steps to ensure his success: "I had to learn to trust my body through trial and error. I needed to develop a system that allowed me to be out for hours. I was always prepared. I always took food, and I took money. It wasn't failsafe: sometimes I came back high, but it was better than the alternative. I now use basal bolus and a continuous glucose monitor for a better effect."

Now, of course, today's athletes are using continuous glucose monitors and newer insulins, but I emphasize that just because you can't afford or access the latest gadgets, it doesn't mean you can't achieve your goals. Yes, being on a pump makes managing the disease easier, as does continuous glucose monitoring technology. However, if you are not on a monitor, you can still achieve great control and outcomes by finding what works for you with what you can access.

Even if you are still using multiple daily injections, the accuracy of today's options is a far cry from yesteryear. As Chris points out, Type 1 diabetes management even at a basic level has come a long way. "I am blown away by people. Any time I talk to someone who had to boil and sharpen their needles and are still around doing great, it amazes me. When I think about the tools that were available to me when I was diagnosed compared to now, those [advances] have really changed how I get to manage this disease." We can all be thankful that we no longer have to sharpen our own needles! (No, that is not a misprint: 50 years ago, diabetics had to do that!)

The takeaway lesson is to make the most of the technology you have—whatever it is—and don't let it be an excuse for not going after your goals.

You will be surprised by how these five simple steps can reduce the subconscious pressure that living with Type 1 diabetes creates. We often struggle not with the disease itself (although that too can be trying), but more so the stress associated with managing it. People online frequently share how they are always thinking about their disease. Take the advice of the neuroscientists who study this field and get your thoughts out of your brain and onto paper. This habit will allow your brain to relax and think about other more important things—such as how you are going to make your first million dollars or go on the dream vacation you've always wanted.

CHAPTER AT A GLANCE

- Small one percent efforts add up over time to produce big results.

- The brain is not as efficient as multitasking as you may think. Focus on one task at a time to achieve great results.

- The brain does not do well at remembering everything. Get it down on paper.

- If you want to create more time, create systems to organize your life.

- A planner is a must if you want to make sure your energy is focused on the right project.

- Planning your time ensures the things that are most important to your progress get the appropriate amount of time.

- If you want to worry less, put the problems on paper and out of your brain.

CHAPTER 8

WHEN THINGS JUST AREN'T CLICKING

When things aren't adding up in your life, start subtracting.
—Brian Tracy

As those of you reading this book can probably attest, the diagnosis of Type 1 diabetes and the health care support that follows can range from awesome to darn right lackluster. Stories abound on the Internet of misdiagnoses, delayed consultations, and Type 1 diabetics started on Type 2 diabetic drugs.

When Chris Angell got his diagnosis of diabetes, the aspiring entrepreneur did not start with a health care team that was meeting his needs, to put it mildly. Chris's Type 1 diabetes began to show on a ski trip. Suddenly feeling very thirsty, he proceeded to guzzle a Gatorade at the bottom of the ski run he was on. By the time he got to the top of the chair lift, he needed to go to the bathroom. Soon he was only skiing the run that had a drink at the bottom and a bathroom at the top. His friends were wondering why Chris was suddenly fascinated with one ski run given that a whole mountain was there to be skied!

The next morning, Chris woke so hungry he consumed a whole pack of hotdogs by himself! His girlfriend (now wife) worked in health care and knew that for a 6' 6" guy who used to weigh 190 pounds and now weighed just 160 pounds, with an insatiable thirst and an unusual hunger for hotdogs, Type 1 diabetes was a definite possibility. Chris recalls, "My family doctor told me that everyone thinks they have diabetes and tried to give me an appointment in three weeks. I had to insist on coming in immediately, and when I was tested I was in the high 300s. I got sent back home on Metformin [a drug for the treatment of Type 2 diabetes] and nothing had changed. I was getting weaker and still losing weight. The doctor's response was to double the dose of Metformin, which obviously had no effect. Finally, I was started on a basal and then a bit later some fast-acting insulin. I finally felt good."

Eight months after this initial diagnosis, Chris finally saw an endocrinologist. He had been given the name of a leading endocrinologist in Washington, but his appointment was rescheduled twice. He learned the endocrinologist had chosen to attend a corporate financial get-together rather than meet his commitment as Chris's care provider. Chris realized that the situation needed changing and set about finding someone more in tune with his needs. "As a result of the delay in medical care, I had protection against the scary parts of the diagnosis. No one told me what I couldn't or shouldn't do. My uncle basically said I could do anything I wanted to, and I took that at face value. As the honeymoon wore off and I started reading about the risks, I didn't need to learn that things were still possible, but rather, that it was more serious than I had thought."

Of course, many health care professionals have made amazing differences to those living with and managing the disease. People often forget that as well trained and smart as doctors are, they are also human. The styles and approaches that work well for some patients do not work well for others. Likewise, personality differences and social styles can impact how messages are conveyed and received.

Not everybody has the luxury of finding out who they get on best with by taking personality tests. Nevertheless, people differ, and it is never a good idea to surround yourself with a group of individuals, in your business or in your personal life, who all think like you do. People with different viewpoints may have new ideas to challenge your thinking and question if there might be a better way. When looking at your team, it is important to take this factor into consideration.

If, however, the situation really isn't working, there is no need to stay with a health care team that is not meeting your needs. Seek an alternative viewpoint from someone else and discuss the choices being made. Kerri's perspective as a Type 1 diabetes advocate summarizes this idea perfectly: "It is important to advocate for yourself. No one is going to do it better than you. Call your insurance company and ask for what you need to achieve that goal. Patients sometimes feel steamrolled by their doctors. If what they suggest doesn't work for them, then they need to speak up and find other ways to achieve the same goal. They can challenge. Doctors are just people. They are not magicians, and it helps when people realize this."

Sir Steve was more fortunate when it came time to work with his endocrinologist. "When I got the diagnosis of diabetes, I thought my rowing career was over. I knew no one who was rowing at this level with diabetes. I figured, I will walk in there and hear the news and that will be it." Ian Gallen, Sir Steve's endocrinologist, had other ideas. He saw no reason why, with some careful management, Sir Steve shouldn't be able to compete at the Olympics. This chance referral resulted in history being made.

Sir Steve explains, "I was at a health care professionals' meeting after the Olympics, with my wife and endocrinologist, and we were doing a presentation. When it came time for questions, an endocrinologist in the crowd said, 'You know, you are very lucky to achieve what you did.' I thought, 'That's a bit cheeky,' but then the endocrinologist said, 'If I or many others had been managing you, your rowing career would have ended on your first visit with us. You were very lucky to have Ian, who saw what was possible.' I then understood how important it was to have the right people with you."

Likewise, Sébastien also needed to find a team of health care professionals willing to support his dream. Climbing Everest would require knowledge of his energy and insulin requirements to keep him as stable as possible. Sébastien asked around until he found health care providers willing to support his dream.

Changing what is not working applies not only to the others on your team: looking inward and trying different approaches can also help in achieving success. By embracing experimentation and making mistakes that you learn from (have I made this point enough already?), you can adapt your approach to something that works better. It is okay to get things wrong.

Athletes might tinker with the type of glucose they eat. If that doesn't help their performance, the next time they might try different insulin settings. Others may experiment with different types of food. (I know that for me, pizza and rice are some of the hardest foods to keep my glucose under control). The point isn't to try to avoid challenges, but rather, once you find them, to remove and replace them with alternatives.

If you are worried about negative consequences from making a mistake, then form a contingency plan to safeguard against them. Sir Steve took glucose drinks in the boat in case he had made a mistake with his insulin and energy requirements. This extra preparation allowed him to experiment with his training and his disease while managing the potential pitfalls.

As Kerri points out, even someone who has years of experience dealing with a challenge such as Type 1 diabetes has to keep an open mind. "I don't consider myself a role model as it gives the impression I have it figured out. This disease can trick you, but it is being open to trial and error that gives you the longevity." With every new skill one learns, there is always an opportunity for mistakes to happen. Inevitably, some can be rather funny if viewed with the right mindset.

I include here some of the amusing stories those I interviewed were kind enough to share. In finding humor in hardship, my intention is not to belittle any challenges you have gone through, nor am I suggesting you should laugh at something that has caused you pain. However, each of the interviewees was more than willing to share a story that they now look back on and laugh about.

To be fair, I will also share a story of my own to illustrate that we all have moments where this disease can get the better of us. In the early years of our courtship, my now wife and I began living together. Like some diabetics, I gave her a slimmed down version of what to expect when dating me, such as what glucagon was used for and why she should call an ambulance if, for some reason, I could not be woken.

I did not mention, however, that hypoglycemia could result in erratic behavior. On one occasion, having arrived home from a long day at work, I began to chat with my wife to be. Noticing that I no longer seemed to be making sense, she suggested I drink some orange juice. Starting to feel the effects of hypoglycemia, my rather sugarless brain processed this kind and astute gesture as her attempting to poison me! I promptly accused her and spent half an hour trying to fight her valiant attempts to get me to drink it. The more she tried, the more I was convinced it was poison.

After I finally came to my senses, I realized the fool I had been. After several days of explaining why things had gone the way they had, I was able to convince her that I was not, in fact, crazy. Thankfully, I am now married to this very understanding woman and no longer fight her efforts to help me on the rare occasions it happens.

As mentioned earlier, Kerri is a joy to talk to thanks to her open and self-deprecating nature. One story she was willing to share with readers of this book is the time a low glucose event resulted in what she now calls her most embarrassing diabetes moment. Her boyfriend at the time had needed to call emergency services to help Kerri get her glucose levels back up. Her dangerously low levels meant that the usually polite and extremely agreeable Kerri was no longer available; she was seemingly a different person. As Kerri tells it, "I had a really belligerent hypoglycemic event, and because I wasn't responding to my boyfriend's instructions and was nearing being unconscious, he called the ambulance. Three guys show up and are really big and strong. Not being quite with it, I called them all a bunch of fat #$&*s while they were trying to help me! I had to go back and apologize a few days later as I felt so bad."

Clearly, Type 1 diabetes is hard to manage no matter who you are. Successful diabetics like Kerri realize that these occurrences are but a moment in time, something to reflect on and laugh about. Life is too short to be embarrassed by this disease. Realizing that we have all had our moments in managing this condition makes us human.

Remember, too, that not everyone's diabetes behaves the same way. Some have found that these circumstances are less likely to occur due to the control they have managed to attain and their recognition of the danger before it occurs. Sir Steve's funny moment illustrates this to a tee—literally. Sir Steve had found that through careful management and testing, he was able to learn quickly how his body responded to his efforts and the insulin he was taking. Interestingly, his second-worst hypoglycemic event did not occur in the boat but rather on the golf course.

Having finished his training in the morning, he, his partner Sir Matthew Pinsent, and the team doctor decided a round of golf was in order. At the clubhouse, he had been told that the halfway house on the course was open. The three set off, with Sir Steve feeling secure in the knowledge that if any issues were to present themselves, they could always grab a quick bite to eat at the halfway point. Of course, the halfway house was closed, and as anyone with Type 1 diabetes can relate, it was the one time that Sir Steve had an issue relating to hypoglycemia.

Sir Steve remembers, "The team doctor looked at me and said, 'We have to go in, don't we?' By this stage, I was definitely feeling lightheaded and agreed that it was probably a good idea. By the time we got back to the clubhouse, I was the worst I'd ever felt. I basically ate half the clubhouse's food before I came right, I was that hungry and that low. I felt pretty ropey for a good 24 hours, and prior to that situation I had never experienced it. It was really a good learning curve for me to go through, so I knew that I didn't want to experience that again."

What the above experience illustrates is that insulin-controlled diabetes, no matter how well managed, can still catch one unawares. Sir Steve had informed those around him of his condition and the potential problems, so when trouble started brewing they were able to do something about it. Furthermore, Sir Steve used the experience as a lesson to better arm himself against future occurrences rather than as something to fear.

Sharing our hypoglycemia stories can help others to understand what to look out for and help us manage should we ever find ourselves in a situation out of our control. Obviously, the goal is never to be needing the help in the first place, but by sharing our stories, we move closer to acceptance and understanding from those around us.

My interviewees also shared some insight on how to approach Type 1 diabetes management, which I include in this chapter to give some perspective. Their suggestions are by no means the be all and end all, and they should not be used without the guidance of medical professionals. In gathering these thoughts, I asked the following question of my interviewees: What advice would you give your younger self and new diabetics that you wish you had known when you were first diagnosed?

Kerri Sparling said, "For those that are going through diagnosis or burnout, I want them to realize there is a life after diabetes. You can still love, laugh, drink. You not robbed of who you are. There is just something extra that you have to do to keep being you. In terms of burnout, I think about just whittling things down into little pieces. The big picture of diabetes is very overwhelming. If I am dealing with not wanting to do the whole picture of testing, carb counting, exercising, I will just focus on one part until I have it nailed. I then move on to the next part. If I can't get that locked in, then I will reach out to the team, who is there to help me."

Kerri's reflections on when she was first diagnosed will, I hope, ease the pressure we put on ourselves with regards to our future. "If I could tell my seven-year-old self something now, it would be to *relax*. It is going to be okay. Your life isn't going to be compromised. You can still have the same pleasures and enjoyment, but you just might have to work a little bit harder to get them."

Sir Steve Redgrave answered, "Communication. You get all this information at one time. From the patient's point of view, ask questions. If you don't get the answers, keep asking questions. If you are a health care professional, don't take it for granted that patients know what you know. We are normal people just like everybody else. We have good days and bad days. There are problems that are put in your path of trying to achieve anything. The outcome is how you respond. The people who I surrounded myself with taught me to keep the freshness of mind that diabetes has to live with me—and not the other way around."

Sir Steve's other gem was his approach to his diabetes management. "If you are a non-diabetic, your body is testing all the time. Testing 10 times a day was just a tiny percentage, but that is as near as it was to what my body was doing before. When you lead a stressful lifestyle, every day, every situation is different. In those early days, I was logging it on an A4 sheet and comparing it to the training. That is why I have trained myself to test as much as I do to get information. The most in control moment in time I could have complete control is when I was in bed asleep. That is where I strive for perfection."

Kayla Brown said, "At first I was strict with myself. I didn't give myself much freedom and beat myself up about non-perfect sugars. Over time I realized there were variances. I do resets every day to try something new to get the best out of it. Diabetes no longer controls my life."

"I really set myself back when I didn't pay attention to my care," Jeff Collins answered. "It is so significant that I have put it into my wedding vows to my new wife. To my younger self I would simply say, 'PAY ATTENTION.'"

Sébastien Sasseville advised, "For the first few years, I was trying to beat my diabetes. It worked, but it was exhausting. After that I realized that I needed to live with it and not fight it. The way I look at it, there is a guy in my living room called diabetes. I can't kick him out, so I might as well get along with it. You don't have to like it, but you have to do it."

Phil Southerland commented, "I would tell my younger self to go with your gut and don't give up. There were a lot of times when things almost didn't work out for me, but I just had to go with it. At 18, that's when I needed the confidence to say, 'You never win if you don't risk losing.'"

In a funny side note, after the interview Phil emailed me and offered another piece of advice that I had to include for its simplicity and wisdom: "Listen to your mother, and listen to your wife. They are right (most of the time). And whatever you do, always do it for the right reason. Do it with honesty and integrity."

As the author of this book and someone who has lived with the disease since I was two (I was born in 1974), my advice is simple. This disease is hard. You will have days when you think you have it mastered only to have one of the worst days of your life the next day. But you are not facing it alone, and don't think we are not all fighting our personal battles, even though on the surface it looks like we have it all worked out. Your last A1c is not your current one. The one bad blood sugar does not ruin the work you took to get the 10 great ones. Focus on what you are doing right, try to repeat it, and learn from the mistakes that are not getting you what you want. This is your life, and you should go after everything you have ever dreamed of, Type 1 diabetes or otherwise!

CHAPTER AT A GLANCE

- Doctors are human, and each has his or her own personality and philosophy. Find one who supports your dreams and goals but also, as importantly, challenges you.
- Outcomes that are not to your liking are simply feedback on the efforts you have been using to achieve your goal.
- Mistakes and challenges are inevitable. Remove things that are not working and try something different to see if it brings a better outcome.
- The approach that works for one may not work for all. Don't be afraid to individualize your options.
- Type 1 diabetes is going to throw you some curve balls. Learning to laugh at the situation helps others want to talk about the challenges more openly.
- You are not alone in managing this disease or dealing with your "uncomfortable situations."
- Hindsight is 20/20, as they say. Embracing some of the funnier moments that occur due to diabetes can give you some entertaining stories for campfire sharing.

CHAPTER 9

WHY CHALLENGES GIVE AS MUCH AS THEY TAKE

Someday, everything will make perfect sense.
So for now, laugh at the
confusion, smile through the tears, be strong and keep
reminding yourself
that everything happens for a reason.
—John Mayer

Ray Dalio, one of the world's richest and most successful entrepreneurs and investors, says in his biography, "If you are not evolving, then you are dying."[31]

On face value, this perspective seems rather extreme, but on diving deeper into his sentiment, Dalio provides context to illustrate that this statement is applicable to any situation—including diabetes. "I keep the pain in perspective," he says, "knowing that I will get through these setbacks and that most of my learning will come from

---

[31] Ray Dalio, *Principles: Life and Work* (New York: Simon and Schuster, 2017).

82

reflecting on them. I have largely gotten past the pain of my mistake and instead enjoy the pleasure that comes from learning from it."

Naturally, Type 1 diabetes has its downsides. I am sure, given the choice, that anyone with the diagnosis would prefer not to have it. However, with every downside there is the potential for an upside. The trick is not to focus on the negative aspects; instead, look for the positives. If you keep this philosophy front of mind, then diabetes is an excellent teacher when it comes to gaining skills.

For Chris Angell, diabetes got him in touch more deeply with his humanity. He says, "[Type 1 diabetes] has given me an awareness and a compassion in terms of judging other people on where they are health wise and appearance wise. As a result of the life I have lived and the people I have met, I realize that their existence is more than what is under their immediate control. Now I am more inclined to think there is more to everyone's story."

Likewise, when Meredith and Kayla created something together from the diagnosis of Type 1 diabetes, it also gave back on a more functional level. For Meredith, "My diagnosis taught me so much. I was always responsible, but now I am more prepared and organized. I found that I am so much healthier than before as I am more aware of what I am eating and focusing on."

And for Kayla, Type 1 diabetes opened up a whole new world of possibility that she had never before considered: "When I was diagnosed, I realized there was so much out there to do. The constant support I have received has been my life-changing moment. It made me realize I wanted to help. In turn, it opened my eyes to taking care of myself and realizing how fragile life is. Once someone is diagnosed with something, that's when they actually start living. Diabetes has given me responsibility and the opportunity to help my community."

In terms of other more functional aspects, Type 1 diabetes provides unique access to resources in the medical system. Having access to a dietician doesn't necessarily need to be focused only on diabetes, for example. If you are an athlete or are trying to get to an ideal weight, these clinicians are qualified to assist. Don't allow yourself to get trapped into seeing just a small part of what is being offered.

This advice goes for life in general. With a bit of research, Type 1 diabetics can find scholarships offered by clinics or communities to attend university. Organizations offer awards for living with the disease for over 25, 50, and 75 years.[32] Communities such as Connected in Motion offer the chance to discover the great outdoors with other like-minded Type 1 diabetics and their families.

If you are an aspiring athlete, you can now be part of a sports team thanks to our featured role model Phil Southerland and Team Novo Nordisk. If you don't quite make the cut for this elite squad, Team Type 1 is on the cycling program Zwift and has a Facebook page.[33]

The most common benefit, as mentioned by all the people interviewed, is that Type 1 diabetes gives back in the potential connections with others living with the disease. That has been my experience as well. Diabetes gave Phil access to his life's purpose, but more importantly, it connected him to how his actions were affecting his outcomes. "Diabetes gave me the drive to change the world. It gave me awareness of the body. It's never lied to me. If I gave the right amount of insulin for my food, I got a good result. If I didn't, it would let me know."

But not everyone sees diabetes as a skills trainer. Kerri Sparling feels that with or without Type 1 diabetes, her drive for success and making a difference would still be there. "I don't give diabetes much credit. I like to think I would be all these things whether I had the disease or not." She concedes, however, that diabetes has "given me perspective on little things, such as if I have the inconvenience of something like a flat tire. I have a better concept of what the big things really are thanks to living with this disease."

Perhaps the best person to illustrate how Type 1 diabetes can bring a change in focus and approach is the person who resisted it the longest—Jeff Collins: "The skill I learned is body awareness, and ironically, I am now super focused on injections, testing, and doctors' appointments."

---

[32] In Canada, Novo Nordisk gives out a limited-edition print of *The Banting House* to those who have lived with Type 1 diabetes for over 50 years. The endocrinologist must contact Novo Nordisk and fill out an application form. Lilly offers a Diabetes Journey Award for people who have lived with Type 1 diabetes for 10, 25, 50, or 75 years. You or your caregiver team can submit an application online: http://lillydiabetes.com/lilly-diabetes-journey-awards.aspx. Joslin has a program open to anyone who has had insulin-dependent diabetes for 25, 50, 75, or more years. You do not have to be a Joslin patient to apply, but some documentation of diagnosis is necessary: http://www.joslin.org/medalist/apply_now.html.

[33] See for example https://www.facebook.com/groups/RaceT1/.

I encourage you to accept that you now have this disease. No amount of anger or frustration will change this fact. What every person in this book conveyed to me was that Type 1 diabetes taught them something about themselves. Diabetes has valuable lessons to offer, and if you apply those lessons to other parts of your life, it may change your outcome as you pursue your goals. It can make you more disciplined, persistent, big-picture oriented, time aware—you name it! It isn't all bad, but sometimes you have to go looking to discover the good.

"Don't forget," advises Sébastien Sasseville, "that diabetes also gives you things that others don't get from having the disease. For me, it's knowledge of my limits. I think one of the things I am most thankful for is that usually when we face obstacles, they come and go. The point with diabetes is it never goes away. The way you look at obstacles, it now becomes a lifestyle, a philosophy. It allows us to never forget the approach we use so we can apply it to other situations."

Now, at the risk of upsetting those who think it's all bad, I have created (drum roll please, and cue the loud, echoing voice)—

THE TOP 10 ADVANTAGES OF LIVING WITH TYPE 1 DIABETES

1. You get some great life skills. Yeah, I know, it's a lifelong condition that requires lots of patience, persistence, and strength of will to manage. Hang on a sec . . . that sounds a lot like qualities of extremely successful people. There you have it.

2. You can eat candy and not feel guilty. The caveat is that it should be to treat a low blood sugar, but in any case, eating glucose sure tastes good even if it is because your sugars are not perfect.

3. You can make a career out of the condition. Just by talking the language of diabetes every day, you will be more familiar with medical terminology than the average Joe. This gives an advantage in any health care–related job and in biology-type subjects at school.

(For the record, I got an A+ in exercise physiology at university four years running—just saying.)

4. It teaches you to be a healthier person. Managing the condition results in carefully tracking food and exercise. By having this focus, you naturally tend to make better lifestyle choices. Result: better physique, better health.

5. You earn more credit card points for free. This one is specific to those with private health insurance (sorry if you don't have any). Because plans cover most supplies, if you purchase using your credit card and then reclaim the money, you end up getting that fancy holiday sooner!

6. You get served on an airplane first. This one is perhaps my favorite. On long-haul flights overseas, by letting the airline know that you need a diabetic meal, you get served first. Often the food is better than the regular meal. This perk sure makes up for the scrutiny through security!

7. You can see "hard-to-see" doctors easily. Endocrinologists are some of the hardest specialists to get an appointment with. As a Type 1 diabetic, you can see them more frequently than most and by default be screened for other conditions so they are caught early. Result: a higher standard of health care.

8. You get to have your own dietician to maximize your results. Personal dieticians are expensive! We get them for free. I lost four pounds simply by changing to a turkey foot-long sub instead of a steak and cheese, all thanks to my diabetic dietician—go figure.

9. You are part of a group of rare individuals (around 93 percent of people in the world do not have Type 1 diabetes), which makes you special. I am sure none of us would choose to live with the condition if we could help it, but being part of something that is rare means we get to connect with people on another level. Result: we can make more friends!

10. You will always know the makeup of foods and be reminded of it every day. We are all taught to count carbohydrates at some point. Yes, it gets old real fast, but on the upside, at least you know what's going down your throat. As a case in point, did you know that Coke sold in the U.S. has double the number of carbohydrates of Coke sold in Canada?

CHAPTER AT A GLANCE

- Type 1 diabetes teaches many skills that can help in your life if you look for the lessons.
- Many resources are at your disposal that can be leveraged to improve other areas of your life.
- As you live with diabetes longer, you can access the many recognitions that companies offer.
- Look for diabetes groups to join that could offer you the opportunity to try new things.

CHAPTER 10

THE KEY TO HAPPINESS (EVEN WHEN LIVING WITH DIABETES)

Happiness is not something ready-made.
It comes from your own actions.
—Dalai Lama

Probably the best story I have ever heard related to happiness is about John Lennon, the famous Beatle. On a request from his high school teacher to write about what he wanted to be when he grew up, John wrote, "Happy." When the teacher called him into class and expressed that John had clearly not understood what the project was about, John replied, "You clearly don't understand what life is meant to be about."

Nothing beats the feeling that comes from being happy. For some people living with Type 1 diabetes, happiness is hard to find with any consistency. In this chapter we look a little more closely at happiness, and whether we can do anything to affect the regularity with which we feel this awesome emotion.

Through the study of the human mind, scientists have determined the area of the brain that lights up when people feel happy. In this quest, Matthieu Ricard, a monk who was part of the Dalai Lama's inner circle, was studied. Due to how his brain lit up on examination, he is thought to be the happiest man on the planet. Now the cynics reading this book might argue that unless you test everybody, how can one determine who is the happiest? Without getting too far into the weeds, Ricard was able to access the relevant area of the brain far more than any other person the researchers had studied.

Now why am I discussing a monk in a book about Type 1 diabetes and success? I am certainly not suggesting that you shave your head and begin a vow of silence. I am sharing this story because happiness is something we want out of life and in this message lies an opportunity for us to secure it. What does the world's most studied, happiest man have to say? Featured on the business podcast *Success: How I Did It* in December 2017,[34] Ricard states that the key to happiness is simple: **"By focusing on others and how you can help them, the contribution you make to them is returned in the happiness you feel in your everyday life."**

I placed his answer in bold for a reason. This simple idea is the core of how to achieve both success and happiness in your life—especially if you are living with Type 1 diabetes.

For a real-world example of this concept that doesn't involve diabetes, take Alcoholics Anonymous. Alcoholics who are trying to sober up are most likely to be successful at sobriety if they complete Step 12 of the 12-step program. What is so special about this step, I hear you ask? This step involves removing the focus on oneself by helping someone else to deal with the addiction. Those who do not complete this step are more likely to relapse.

Now, I am sure you are wondering how this information relates to the stories you have read throughout this book. Here's the answer: all the people featured in this book took it upon themselves to help

---

[34] Matthieu Ricard, "How I went from a PhD in genetics to being called 'the happiest man in the world,'" December 22, 2017, in *This Is Success*, produced by Business Insider, podcast, https://itunes.apple.com/ca/podcast/success-how-i-did-it/id1205997729?mt=2 &i=1000398100423.

others. They blogged, they formed their own companies based around helping others, they gave talks to inspire, and they became role models within their communities. Ultimately, they each created value for others. I'm not saying that everyone reading this book needs to adopt the next newly diagnosed diabetic and teach that person "the way." But when you take on a challenge and share it with others, the burden is lessened. The joy of seeing others overcome their challenges is a reward that results in you feeling your life is of value.

Take Kayla, for instance. Not only does she attempt to find the funnier side of the many challenges of Type 1 diabetes to make others feel better, but she also gives back in a meaningful way to teenage girls living with the disease. "All these firsts happen in the teen years, and couple this with diabetes. It is difficult. I want to provide a place where these girls have someone to confide in, to help deal with these challenges." This focus has given Kayla meaning in her life.

After Everest, the Sahara Race, and the Ironman, Sébastien ran across Canada to raise awareness of Type 1 diabetes. For 4,500 miles (7,200 kilometers), he traveled through mountain ranges and across vast prairie fields, traversing terrain that would test the measure of any person and that took Sébastien to some fairly dark places as he battled blisters and exhaustion. When I asked him if he ever thought of giving up, his response gives insight into why this concept of giving back is so important: "Not for a second. I had my dark days both psychologically and physically, but we are not our bad days. The reason I didn't give up was the *purpose* I had in doing this. Interviewing 150 people living with the disease made it possible. The 'what' doesn't matter; it is the 'why' that makes it possible. When your purpose is clear, when the mission is more important than individual success, **when you focus on impact rather than performance, you can access the most incredible fuel there is.** That's the most important advice I have for people."

Similarly, when Chris faces another 12-hour day, overcoming the many challenges of running his business, his motivation comes back to the why. "It's important to think about what you want to do and more importantly the why. It is the *why* that when things are not going right, you have something to pull you through it. Everything we do is based around the fact that we come to our jobs with a lot of compassion. Not just the fact we use the product, but the fact that diabetes is a time-consuming, expensive disease."

It also pays to remember that whatever you are aiming for outside of diabetes, finding your reason for taking on the challenge is a crucial component. It doesn't always need to be for altruistic reasons. Take Sir Steve's final Olympic Games as an example. In the months leading up to the games, Diabetes U.K. thought he would make a great poster boy for the disease. "I said, 'Hang on,'" he laughs, "'let's make sure I win before we promote this. If I lose, it isn't the best story.'"

As it happened, over the next three years Sir Steve and his team members won every race at the world championships bar one. That one loss was due to preparation, not diabetes. By proving to himself he still could beat the world's best, Sir Steve now gives back to the diabetes community by speaking at major events and supporting those chasing their sporting dreams.

Phil and his wife, Dr. Biljana Southerland, have recognized that some Type 1 diabetics are missing not just the latest technology, but also the actual insulin needed to treat the disease. In some developing countries, medication isn't even an option! Together they have developed the Team Type 1 (TT1) Foundation (Phil is the president) to fight for the right to life through a global mission of education, empowerment, and equal access to medicine for everyone affected by diabetes. Phil also gives back with Team Novo Nordisk. At each leg of a race, Phil encourages those living with Type 1 diabetes to meet the team. With a following of over 8 million people, Team Novo Nordisk is one of the largest sports organizations, and the largest diabetic organization, in the world.

You may think that you are just one person and your efforts may not make a difference, but Phil and his wife have shown how one vision, with enough passion behind it, can result in big things for many people.

This book you are reading is a function of this sentiment. If I hadn't thought I would be helping you, the reader, take on a bigger challenge and be inspired to do more with your life, I would not have finished or published this book. Many (many!) times I felt like giving up. It seemed that the stories, as great as they are, were just too hard to write about coherently. But because of the difference I know this information could make to others, I persisted.

This book is a way to help everyone living with Type 1 diabetes learn the lessons that drive success. I must say, it has helped me to feel better about the day to day. I wanted to make sure I also contributed to the bigger picture, to help those struggling to live due to lack of access to medications. That is why I am giving 10 percent of the net proceeds to TT1. By buying this book, you have helped to support TT1's vision of providing insulin to everyone with Type 1 diabetes.

What could you do to make a difference to others? Could you volunteer to help clean up your community? Help at school on a volunteer project? Do you want to raise money for research? I can't tell you what your WHY is. I will leave that to you. But finding the answer is honestly the key to leading a happy and fulfilled life.

CHAPTER AT A GLANCE

- Happiness is an elusive concept, but the key to getting it with more regularity is focusing on helping others achieve their goals.
- When your focus becomes about others, it is easier to get through the tough moments that life throws at you.
- Sébastien Sasseville's advice bears repeating: "When you focus on impact rather than performance, you can access the most incredible fuel there is."

ACTION PLAN

The distance between your dreams and reality
is called action.
—Author unknown

It's your turn to act on the words you have read.

As we have covered in the preceding chapters, a dream without action is just a dream. This chapter provides some real-world stepping stones to help you begin your journey to greatness. This action plan is by no means a comprehensive list, but it will help you begin your quest to achieve your goals and overcome the challenges of Type 1 diabetes. Use it as a starting point to get the ideas and plans into place that will help you move forward.

By beginning with the end in mind, you can map out a journey of what is possible. If you feel you could never be prepared enough to be ready to start, the best way forward is to begin with something and then work it out as you go along. History is littered with examples of those who did just that and ended up achieving amazing things.

The Beatles played music because they enjoyed it and wanted to make money over the summer. They travelled to Germany, playing in seedy bars, testing out what worked and what didn't. From all accounts they were not amazing players, but over time, by leaning into it and not hesitating to play in less glamorous surroundings, they became the legends they are today.

Kerri Sparling didn't become a computer whiz before starting her blog *Six Until Me*; she simply started writing. The result is a career in media, the ability to stay home with her daughter and son, a book deal, sponsorships, and paid writing gigs for many online sites. All this transpired because she hoped to connect with others.

Jeff Collins didn't know how to be a radio broadcaster, but that lack of knowledge didn't stop him from taking his first step. The young Jeff went out, knocked on a few doors, and kept making inquiries until he got a roadmap of where to go, resulting in a career hosting the prestigious drive time segment, one which lasted him until he retired.

Phil Southerland came up with the notion of an international team of Type 1 racers during an undergraduate management course at university. He had no idea if it was possible, just that it was something that had to be tried. His idea was so crazy that others told him it couldn't be done. Rather than accept these warnings, Phil leaned into it, and what began with a $400 donation from an anonymous guy at Starbucks is now a major cycling force sponsored by one of the world's biggest insulin manufacturers, Novo Nordisk.

Sir Steve did not know he wanted to be an Olympic rower when he first seized the opportunity to row a boat at high school. He just thought it might be fun. As each year progressed and the team of boys he was a part of did well, they took their skill and tested it against the next challenge. By age 16, he realized he had a shot at becoming a world champion and then really started to focus. The point? You are not born a champion; you make yourself one. If you have a dream, start trying to achieve it. That is what this chapter is all about.

As we discussed earlier in the book, luck is where opportunity meets preparation. Each of these individuals, upon realizing what they wanted to achieve, set about gaining the skills and taking the necessary steps to make it happen. You can do this, too.

To give you a personal example of the process in action, I want to share with you how this book came about. Having had two close friends diagnosed with Type 1 diabetes, I noticed how hard it was for them to come to terms with the diagnosis. I realized there was nothing that I could reference to help inspire them. Knowing nothing about writing a book, or how to get access to famous people, I simply started inquiring. Once a few interviews had taken place, the next step was learning how I could get this book published so you could enjoy it. Podcasts helped me out immensely.

Before I published this book, I thought that I should maybe do a practice book so that I could make a few mistakes. The result is *North Island: New Zealand Travel Secrets*, which I published on Amazon. I took each of these steps one at a time to reach the goal of getting this book into your hands. By writing down the goal and working back from it, breaking it into individual steps, it no longer seemed as daunting.

The pages that follow are *one* way of creating a vision and goals, just as all the people featured in this book, once upon a time, imagined. Do it the way that works for you, but when creating a vision, think as big and bright as possible. Your vision should inspire you and be specific.

Form a vision of what the perfect life would look like for you. Write down goals that, if achieved, would start moving you towards the vision you are creating. A big vision doesn't happen overnight and is made up of achieving many little goals. The first step is focusing on the first small goal. The small goal is the first step in getting you to where you want to go. As Daniel Levitin points out in *The Organized Mind*, the brain gets positive reinforcement as each mini task is completed.

Below is a worksheet for you to make a start. If you are like me, you probably will hear a little voice in your head saying to come back to this later, but don't. Your little voice probably also suggested that this book should be kept in pristine condition. I wrote it to be written in, so get a pen! Write down the first major vision that comes to mind and do the work. You will be surprised where this process will lead you over the coming years.

MY VISION

Insert or glue a picture or pictures that represent what you want to achieve. Print or copy this page and stick it somewhere you will see it every day.

To achieve your vision, it needs to be backed up by goals. Several studies looking into the importance of goals have shown their impact. In a controversial Harvard study from 1979,[35] students were asked if they wrote down goals. Of the class, just 13 percent said that they had written down their goals, and only three percent had written them down *along with a firm plan* on how to attain them.

When the researchers followed up 10 years later, the 13 percent who had written down their goals were making twice as much as the others. The three percent who had written down both their goals and a plan were making *10 times* the amount of the class.

In another study, *The Huffington Post* reported that Dr. Gail Matthews looked at 267 people from a variety of backgrounds. She showed that of this group, the people who had written down their goals were 42 percent more likely to achieve them than those who hadn't.[36] Even if you don't believe these findings to be accurate, try it out to prove me wrong and see what can happen.

Setting goals can be a very good kind of addiction. According to Simon Sinek, who wrote the book *Leaders Eat Last*,[37] writing goals down and achieving them releases dopamine, which in turn gives a feeling of pleasure. Through this mechanism, one can constantly be moving forward and feeling good about it, just because of the way the brain likes to be rewarded.

A good goal is measurable and specific. It has a date by which it will be achieved. It has as much detail as possible, along with the feelings that will be associated with achieving it.

Once your goal is in writing, write down the steps you will need to take to complete it. This is another trick that those who have tasted success know well. By breaking down a bigger goal into smaller, more manageable pieces, the task no longer seems as daunting, and you increase the chances that you too will taste success.

On completing the goal statement and steps, write down the obstacles you expect to face and what role diabetes may or may

---

[35] The study is controversial because no one is sure if it really happened; if so, it was conducted before the time of robust record keeping. For an interesting discussion on the topic, see https://www.wanderlustworker.com/the-harvard-mba-business-school-study-on-goal-setting/.

[36] Mary Morrissey, "The Power of Writing Down Your Goals and Dreams," *The Huffington Post*, December 6, 2017, https://www.huffingtonpost.com/marymorrissey/the-power-of-writing-down_b_12002348.html.

[37] Simon Sinek, *Leaders Eat Last: Why Some Teams Pull Together and Others Don't* (New York: Penguin, 2014).

not play. For each obstacle you write down, think of what steps you could take to minimize its impact. By doing this planning, you will no longer be distracted by the obstacle, and you will increase your chance of success.

A great example of this technique is Sébastien's climb on Mount Everest. He knew that at a certain altitude, his tester no longer worked accurately, and his pump was not proven to be safe. Knowing that hypoglycemia or diabetic ketoacidosis would end his ability to summit, he came up with a plan to get around the obstacle and still achieve his goal. By learning to listen to his body when training for his climb, he knew roughly how he was doing with respect to his glucose when he was unable to test on his attempt at the summit. As we know, Sébastien achieved this feat and is now recognized as the first Canadian Type 1 diabetic to summit Mount Everest, in part because he adopted a process to manage obstacles.

Likewise, Sir Steve knew that despite all the training prior to the Olympics, he did not want to sap his mental strength with an underlying doubt about his sugar going low in the gold medal race. He didn't try to forget about it and hope for the best as he lined up at the start line in the 2000 Olympic coxless four final. Instead, he had taken precautionary steps in case something went wrong: "Just before the race, I was thinking, 'What happens if I have problems today? What happens if I go low today?' I decided to get two sachets of sugar from the canteen and tape them to the inside of the boat, just in case. I forgot I had put them there as I didn't need them during the race or after. When the boat came back to England, it was placed in the River and Rowing Museum complete with the sachets that were discovered on its arrival!"

Thanks to Sir Steve, we now all have an inside piece of knowledge that, as a member of the Diabetes Club, you can truly appreciate.

The trick to living with Type 1 diabetes isn't to pretend that it doesn't have a role in your life, your significant other's life, or your child's life. Rather, by using the idea of proactively finding strategies to address the challenge, you increase the likelihood of your success (whatever that looks like for you). By planning the steps to address it, you are one further step ahead in your journey.

So, if reaching your goals and achieving what you set out to do before Type 1 diabetes entered your life is something you are interested in, I strongly encourage you to complete the next section (even if you humor me, as I know how much effort this is).

Write out your answers to the statements below and insert your information in the sections that are underlined. Even if you class yourself as the world's biggest cynic on this sort of thing, I know that if you try it and look back on it after a year, you will be surprised by the results and by how much closer you are to your goal. (I say this as I used to be that cynic.)

Furthermore, it is important to remember *why* you want to go after your goal in the first place. When I asked Sir Steve what kept him going, he stated, "The most important thing is to enjoy what you are doing. You don't have to enjoy every session of every day. That's crazy. Fifty to 75 percent of the time is about right. It will allow you to keep practicing. If you talk to anyone at the top of their field, it is more a passion than a job." His honesty can give any of us a realistic expectation of what might motivate us.

MY GOAL

By _________________________, I have ___________________________.
      [insert date of completion]   [insert what you want to achieve]

As a result of this achievement, I am _________________________.
                          [insert feeling associated with the goal]

I will take the following steps to reach my goal: ___________________.
                               [insert your steps]

I expect the following the challenges to occur: ___________________.
                             [insert your challenges]

I propose the following solutions to manage them: _______________.
                             [insert your solutions]

To achieve this goal, I will need the support of the following people

or organizations: ____.

After setting your amazing goals, you can do one more thing to get ahead. As you might have witnessed in the pregame routines of elite athletes, many will be closing their eyes, talking to themselves. No, these elite athletes are not part of some cult; they are visualizing their success.

Visualization can apply to your life, too. If you are interested in beginning the process of visualizing your goals, one simple method is through guided meditation. Now I know some of you may be thinking I am some sort of quack for making this suggestion (it also explains why I put it at the end, so I at least had half a chance of establishing credibility), but stick with me on this.

Some authorities have suggested that we attract what we think about.[38] I think this concept has some merit if we look a little closer. The human psyche has to deal with so much stimuli that it must screen out many everyday circumstances to avoid becoming overloaded. Consider what happens when you buy a new car. Prior to the purchase, you may never have noticed that color, or that make and model, on the road. After your purchase, however, it is common to notice your make and model all the time. What has changed? The difference is that your subconscious mind is now looking for it, so you in turn notice it.

Where am I going with this discussion?

Visualization, or meditation, provides the mind with an opportunity to slow down and start to notice things. In terms of goals, visualizing and meditating on a specific goal can provide you with ideas you might otherwise not have thought of. They also awaken your subconscious mind to notice opportunities that may help you get to your goal. If you don't believe me, try them and see. You will be amazed at what suddenly "appears" to help you in chasing your dreams when you begin to focus on them. It isn't necessarily that the universe is now conspiring to help you. Rather, your mind notices opportunities that it previously viewed as inconsequential and unimportant and now presents them to you as something you want to know about.

For the next month, I encourage you to meditate about or visualize what you are wanting to achieve (just like the greats in business and sport do) and see what happens. Even if you do it to prove me wrong, I think you will get great value out of the exercise.

---

[38] See for example Rhonda Byrne, The Secret, 10th anniversary ed. (New York: Simon and Schuster, 2016).

CHAPTER AT A GLANCE

- Begin with a vision of what you want your life to be, then set goals that will get you there.
- Writing down goals makes it more likely you will achieve them.
- Visualizing and meditating are not as weird as you might think. They help your subconscious see obvious things that your brain was previously ignoring that might help you.
- Developing an action plan is the first step to getting to where you want to be. It should include finding a way to manage some of the setbacks you may encounter.

CONCLUSION

*Life doesn't require that we be the best, only that we try
our best.*
—H. Jackson Brown, Jr.

I hope that as a result of reading this book, you have at the very least been inspired. This is by no means a manual on how to live your life or what you should do to feel better about the diagnosis of Type 1 diabetes. We are all on our own journeys. The feelings we have about managing this disease are going to vary greatly, as is the ease we find in managing it. You do, however, have choices you can make each day. By making different choices, you can make a huge difference to your outcomes.

You can decide to continue going after your dreams, drawing on the diagnosis as a chance to test yourself, learn to overcome obstacles, and potentially leverage them for a career. Alternatively, you could resign yourself to battling the disease and letting it limit the dreams and aspirations that once inspired you to grow and reach for the stars. Ultimately the choice is yours to make. Realize that whatever your aspirations are, it is 100 percent up to you to make them happen.

The stories featured here are unique to those discussed but are by no means unique to achieving goals. Every successful person in life overcomes an obstacle, a circumstance, or a setback. For you to do the same will involve a growth mindset, a team of people, a vision and a plan for where you want to go, and a willingness to do what it takes to get the job done.

On this note, if you were to ignore that each of the awesome individuals featured here lives with diabetes, and instead focus only on their achievements, the following would be true:

- Phil started a professional cycling team and is attempting to qualify for the Tour de France. He established his team's credibility by winning the Race Across America with a group of elite cyclists and secured sponsorships from major corporations to make it happen.

- Sébastien climbed Mount Everest, raced in the Sahara, ran across Canada to raise awareness of Type 1 diabetes, and completed seven Ironman competitions. Through achieving these goals, he became a paid public speaker that corporations hire to inspire their employees.

- Kerri started a blog that became an Internet sensation, wrote a book, and is a paid health consultant, a recognized thought leader, and a patient advocate.

- Kayla and Meredith put a passion for humor online and created a business in the process. They have used these skills to make a difference to countless individuals struggling to find the lighter side of life.

- Jeff became a popular radio host with a distinguished career, hosting the prime drivetime segment before retiring.

- Chris addressed a need for a faster, better way to take glucose and created a business in the process.

- Sir Steve won five gold medals in consecutive Olympics. For this unique achievement, he was knighted by Her Majesty Queen Elizabeth II in recognition of his contribution to the British kingdom.

Diabetes was not the reason for any of these successes—nor did it stop these remarkable individuals from attempting their dreams, despite not being guaranteed success. The main thing they all have in common is that they started (and persevered). Take your first step now.

I hope you find your strength and look toward what is possible now that I have shown you the path that others have already travelled. The first step to realizing your dreams and aspirations is simply believing it is possible and focusing on that possibility. The next and most important step is taking just one action, seeing what result it produces, and following it up with another.

PAY IT FORWARD

If this book in any way makes a difference to how you view your situation, please don't keep it to yourself. I encourage you to share it with people you know—not for my benefit, but for theirs. Everyone deserves a chance to thrive. This book, and the amazing people in it, may be the difference.

As with any book, discovery usually comes by word of mouth. In today's online world, that's often an online review. If this book has helped to create a brighter future for you or a loved one, I would be grateful if you would spend just two minutes to write a review. It doesn't have to be long; even a few words could go a long way in helping others living with Type 1 diabetes to discover and be inspired by this book.

Most important, I look forward to hearing *your* success stories and hope that someday I might interview you as you make your difference in the world. As you have read, sharing your goals is a stepping stone to realizing your dreams. If after reading this book you are inspired to take on a challenge, let me know specifically what you intend to do.

My email address is type1skillset@gmail.com.
Tim Hoy

APPENDIX: INFO YOU DIDN'T KNOW BUT WERE TOO SCARED TO ASK

I wrote this section to clarify Type 1 diabetes and cover some of the many questions that new diabetics have. To make it easy to read and understand, I have not gone into detail. If you need more in-depth information about these points, discuss them with your doctor.

What is HbA1c, and what is the ideal number based on? HbA1c stands for *glycosylated* (or *glycated*) *hemoglobin*. It is basically a fancy way of indicating how much sugar has been in the blood over a three-month period based on the blood taken from a person's body. The body's red blood cells have a protein called hemoglobin on their surface that binds sugar. Given that a blood cell lives from eight to 12 weeks, the amount of sugar bound to the cell's surface is used to indicate the average level of sugar over its lifespan. A landmark trial known as the DCCT (Diabetes Control and Complications Trial) found that the ideal HbA1c number for a Type 1 diabetic is between six and seven. Participants in that range had the best outcomes in mitigating negative outcomes of having Type 1 diabetes. Lower numbers put Type 1 diabetics at an unacceptable risk of hypoglycemia.

What is insulin, and what does it do? It amazes me that for those of us who have to take insulin to survive, not all of us know exactly what this liquid is that we inject. Insulin is a hormone made by the body's pancreas that regulates the amount of glucose in the blood; it is a transporter molecule that binds glucose and allows it to travel into the body's cells to be used. Those who have Type 1 diabetes don't make enough insulin (due to the islet cells being attacked by the body) or make next to no insulin. To survive, insulin must be injected. Matching the intake of glucose with the amount of insulin allows for the body to maintain a healthy environment for cells to do their jobs. It is the only method that allows sugar to get into the cells. In its absence the body thinks it needs energy and so breaks down fat. The byproduct results in acidic blood, otherwise known as ketoacidosis.

What is the difference between basal and bolus insulin? Every person without diabetes makes insulin. When no food is being consumed, the pancreas releases insulin to keep sugars stable. This is known as the basal rate. In Type 1 diabetics, a basal insulin is a long-acting insulin designed to keep sugars stable when no food is on board. Basal insulins are typically injected once or twice a day. Those on a pump will have a basal rate, which can vary depending on the time of day, and is controlled based on the settings programmed by the user.

When people without diabetes consume food, their pancreas releases extra insulin to respond to the increased amount of energy available. This is known as a bolus insulin. In Type 1 diabetes, this is the insulin we inject just before we eat. We measure how well we estimated by the two-hour post-eating (or post-prandial) blood test we perform.

What are the units of measurement for glucose around the world, and how do I convert them? In the U.S., the unit of measurement for glucose is in milligrams per deciliter (mg/dl). Most other countries use millimols per litre (mmol/L). Neither unit is more accurate than the other, but it can be tricky when reading resources if you are not using the same measurement. To convert from mg/dl to mmol/L, divide by 18. To convert from mmol/L to mg/dl, multiply by 18.

Each region of the world has its ideal range for blood glucose, and doctors may change this range if needed (e.g., a patient suffering from hypoglycemia unawareness). Generally speaking, however, this is what is suggested:

- Fasting glucose (the glucose value when you have not eaten for a long period of time, such as when you first wake up): from 4.0–7.0 mmol/L (72–126 mg/dl).
- Post-prandial glucose (the glucose value after consuming food): from 5.0–10.0 mmol/L (90–180.mg/dl).

The above ranges vary across governing organizations. For simplicity's sake, I have opted to use values from the Canadian Diabetes Association, which are similar to suggestions from the American Diabetes Association and the Joslin Diabetes Center.

What causes blood sugar drops during exercise? Glucose can get from the blood to cells that need it in two ways. One is with the use of insulin (the transporter molecule). The other is through contracting muscles. This is why, when you exercise for a period of time, your body may need less insulin. The glucose uptake in the body is being assisted by your muscles. The change in insulin requirements is influenced by the type, intensity, and duration of the exercise, as well as prior exercise. To say that a process of trial and error is required to get the insulin levels right is an understatement. But as we covered in this book, the more we monitor our bodies, the more understanding we obtain.

What is glucagon, and how does it work? Think of glucagon as being the yin to insulin's yang. Like insulin, it is a hormone. Glucagon's job is to get the liver to secrete its glucose store when there is not enough glucose in the body. Although Type 1 diabetics still make glucagon, the feedback mechanism for its secretion can be impaired, and therefore our ability to secrete glucose through this mechanism when we are low is also impaired. When we are in so much distress that we can no longer eat the necessary grams of carbohydrate, first responders or our significant others will inject this hormone. On being injected with glucagon, the body gets the reserved stores of glucose from the liver released and, more often than not, we recover. We should be sure to eat after getting one of these shots as our bodies need to replace the stores.

Why do I stop being able to function below a certain glucose level? As we all know, low glucose leads to low performance. So, what causes this drop? The brain is a hungry machine. Unlike the rest of the body, it does not require insulin to use glucose. However, if glucose is no longer available due to too much insulin being used to cover food or correcting high sugar, the brain's performance crashes. Without glucose, the brain's ability to control the body starts to decline. At this point we can begin to convulse, become sleepy, or, for those of you who have read chapter 8, accuse our girlfriend of trying to kill us.

How come I get so thirsty when I have a high sugar reading? Thirst, and regularly needing to use the washroom, are two side effects of the body trying to set itself back to baseline. Excess sugar in the blood is removed by the kidneys and is excreted through the urine, which necessitates multiple trips to the loo. As the body tries to get energy by burning fat, ketones start to become a problem. To compensate, the body tries to get rid of these as well. This process results in thirst, as the body now becomes dehydrated.

At a basic level, what is the difference between Type 1 and Type 2 diabetes? Perhaps the biggest annoyance of being a Type 1 diabetic is the assumption by the general public that all diabetics are the same. The number of times I have heard, "You must have been fat as a kid," or "You must have eaten too much sugar as a child" is enough to drive anyone crazy.

That said, here is a simplistic explanation of the difference. Type 1 diabetes is an autoimmune disease characterized by the body attacking its own insulin-producing cells, known as beta cells. Over time, the amount of insulin being produced by these cells declines. This explains why there is a "honeymoon" period in the early stages of diagnosis, during which the body is still making its own insulin. As time goes on, the insulin requirements of Type 1 diabetics will increase. This escalation is not reflective of poor management, but rather the output and function of insulin-producing beta cells decreasing over time. The only effective treatment for Type 1 diabetes is insulin—not nutmeg, not cinnamon, and certainly not dealing with your inner self-worth (as a naturopath tried to inform me recently).

Type 2 diabetes has a much different mechanism. Simply put, the body's ability to use the insulin that is being produced becomes compromised. It is a complex disease that is common in people who are overweight (although not always as evidenced by Sir Steve Redgrave). Treatment starts out by using molecules that treat the body's insulin resistance and imbalance of hormones. As time goes on, the body becomes less effective at making insulin due to the large amounts required. This, in turn, can lead to the need for insulin to help control sugars.

What are the risks of Type 1 diabetes? As the saying goes, knowledge is power. This next answer is not meant to be alarmist; I have included these risks out of love and not to worry you. Several of the interviewees in this book mentioned how their loved ones informed them of the consequences of not maintaining good control. Maintaining good control significantly reduces these risks, and there is no reason why you can't have a healthy, happy life *and* have Type 1 diabetes.

Neuropathy: This is a problem related to nerves. After being exposed to high levels of glucose in the blood, the nerve fibers begin to send signals of pain to the brain, leaving people with sharp pains in their extremities. Over time, the pain receptors can stop functioning, leaving people unable to feel injuries or cuts, which can lead to infections and amputations from these infections.

Infections: Infections take longer to heal if glucose is high in the blood. The immune system becomes less effective at fighting disease. As noted above, neuropathy can result in an infection going unnoticed, which can lead to amputation. Check your toes and feet regularly, and if something isn't healing, see your doctor.

Retinopathy: Poor control over a long period of time can lead to diabetic retinopathy. The small capillaries in the eyes become damaged by excess glucose and "leak" into the field of view. The condition is treatable, using a laser to cauterize the offending vessel, but it must be caught early. Regular check-ups with an optometrist are essential.

Impotence: This is obviously a male-only problem. As with the eyes, blood vessels in the lower extremities become damaged by poor control, resulting in trouble on a very personal level.

ACKNOWLEDGEMENTS

Every book exists thanks to a great team, and this book is no exception. It took me over five years to write. I went through stages where I felt the message I had to share would not resonate with those reading it. At times I wondered if I should even finish. Had it not been for the amazing people in my life, this book would never have made it to print.

My loving family encouraged me to share my passion for making a difference and persevering in securing the stars of Type 1 diabetes. My amazing wife has lived with the challenges of Type 1 diabetes that I have faced and accepted them as her own. Without her, I would never have achieved all that I have, and I certainly would not have finished this book (thanks for reminding me monthly of my goals!). Her reading of my book, and her valuable feedback to make it better, helped me more than she will ever know. My adorable children inspired me to continue to write and always encouraged me to be my best. Your love and acceptance without judgement make everything I do feel worth it.

To my mom and dad, thanks so much for looking past me having Type 1 diabetes and seeing me as the person I am. This view helped me never to let the disease get in the way of chasing my dreams. Mom, you were ahead of your time in helping me own my disease, sometimes pushing me when I didn't want it. I have you to thank for the awesome life I have today, without any complications, despite being diagnosed in 1976.

My thanks and appreciation to all the awesome people I got a chance to interview, who so generously gave their time despite not knowing who I was or how long I would take to write this book. All of you have immense demands placed on your time by those inside and outside the diabetic community. Your graciousness and willingness to contribute have been remarkable. Your stories are inspirational. Your willingness to help get the message out about this book, even when you hadn't heard from me in a number of years, inspired me to continue.

Of course, when writing a book, many errors are made, so to my great editor, Karen Crosby from Editarians, I thank you for your patience and speedy work, which has allowed me to get this book into the hands of all of us living with Type 1 diabetes.

Finally, and most importantly, to those who have bought and read this book: I wrote it for you, so that you no longer think your dreams and aspirations are impossible. I hope you realize that success is a function of your commitment and attitude. You will always have an extra challenge compared to those living without Type 1 diabetes, but this need not stop you in chasing your dreams. I thank you for making my dream possible by buying this book, so that I could be an author who makes a difference to others.

ABOUT THE AUTHOR

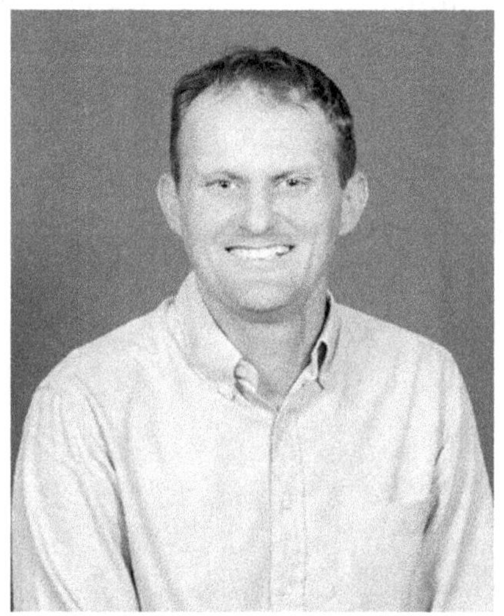

Tim Hoy was born in New Zealand in 1974. He was diagnosed as a Type 1 diabetic at the age of two. Throughout his years of living with the disease, he has seen many changes around the management of Type 1 diabetes and has had many opportunities to meet people living with the disease.

Always wanting to test himself, he represented the province of Waikato in field hockey in high school. He then attended Otago University on New Zealand's South Island, where, after taking up rowing for the first time, he went on to win a gold medal in the 1996 university men's novice eights. He graduated with an honors degree in physical education with a major in biomechanics in 1997.

Wanting to see the world, he became a ski instructor in 1997, traveling to Canada on a student work abroad program at Mt. Norquay, near Banff, Alberta. He relocated to Australia to become an associate producer at Fox Sports before moving permanently to Canada in 2009, where he now works and lives with his wife and two children.

Tim's mother and brother have both lived with diabetes, giving him unique insight into how different personalities find a way that works for them to manage the disease and live the lives they've always dreamed.

Books and other resources on Type 1 diabetes usually focus on challenges and hardships, but when interviewing some bright stars from the world of diabetes, Tim realized they shared many traits. People and their attitudes make the difference; Type 1 diabetes plays a very secondary role in these people's lives. Tim wanted to share their stories in a manner that would allow others to move forward to live the life they had always imagined before diabetes came along.

This journey has culminated in *Tested*.